# Admission Register of
# Central State Hospital
# Milledgeville, Georgia
# 1842–1861

# Admission Register of Central State Hospital Milledgeville, Georgia 1842–1861

Paul K. Graham

The Genealogy Company
Decatur, Georgia

Admission Register of Central State Hospital, Milledgeville, Georgia, 1842–1861




Published by
The Genealogy Company
P.O. Box 1091
Decatur, Georgia 30031

Paperback Edition

ISBN-13: 978-0-9755312-8-0
ISBN-10: 0-9755312-8-X

LCCN: 2011926235


For more information, visit the author's website:
www.pkgraham.com/centralstate

# Contents

# Introduction

This book contains the admission record for the first 888 patients admitted to the Central State Hospital in Milledgeville, Georgia. The hospital, the state's first mental institution, was authorized in 1837 and opened to patients at the end of 1842. Each patient record begins with a list of basic facts, with their name, county of origin, age, marital status, and other facts depending on the particular patient. The introductory information is followed by a description of symptoms that led the patient to the hospital, along with possible causes of illness. Records end with dates of admission then those for elopement (escape), dismission, or death. The number by each individual is the sequential patient number given in early admission records.

At its founding, the hospital was called the Georgia Lunatic Asylum. It began on a forty-acre campus, located south of Milledgeville near Midway, which has since expanded to 1,750 acres. The first superintendent was Dr. David Cooper, who was also one of the hospital trustees. The staff during the 1840s included the superintendent, steward, matron, watchman, two attendants, and two servants. Cooper served to 1845 when he was dismissed and replaced as superintendent by Dr. Thomas A. Green. Green instituted numerous significant changes, among them: abolishing forms of restraint, hiring white nurses (instead of slaves), and instituting a system of classification among patients. He served until 1874. The institution's name was changed to the Georgia State Sanitarium in 1898, then to the Milledgeville State Hospital in 1929, and finally to Central State Hospital in 1967.

Three indexes can be found at the end of this book. The first includes every name, both patient's and close contacts referenced in the records. The second index lists causes of commitment. Due to the nature of the records, a cause was not listed for many patients. No effort to index every noted symptom was attempted. The third index includes every location mentioned in the records. Place names with no state are in Georgia. Out-of-state locations are noted.

No major changes were made during the transcription process. Personal names were transcribed as they appear in the record. Where place names were misspelled in minor ways, they were changed without note (Bullock to Bulloch). Brackets [] were used to note major changes, illegible text, and clarifications. Throughout the text, minor changes were made to improve ease of reading; this included adding and removing commas, as well as changing capitalized common nouns to lower case.

Copies of the records transcribed in this book are available on microfilm at the Georgia Archives. Additional Central State Hospital records available on microfilm include admission records through the 1920s, registers of individuals buried in the hospital cemeteries, and operations records of the institution. For more records created since 1924, contact the hospital directly. Medical privacy laws apply.

Central State Hospital
620 Broad Street, Milledgeville, Georgia, 31062
(478) 445-4128
www.centralstatehospital.org

**Apoplexy**: "Sudden paralysis and coma from effusion and extravasation of blood or serum into the brain or spinal cord." (Stroke, cerebral hemorrhage.)

**Catamenia**: "Menstruation, or the menses." (Many women were committed at the onset of menopause, recorded as "cessation of catamenia." Also referred to as the "critical" time of life.)

**Cutaneous**: "Pertaining to the skin."

**Delirium tremens**: "A variety of acute insanity marked by delirium with trembling and great excitement, and attended by anxiety, mental distress, sweating, and precordial pain. It is caused by abuse of alcoholic stimulants or, more rarely, by opium."

**Dyspepsia**: "Impairment of the power or function of digestion."

**Epilepsy**: "A chronic functional disease characterized by fits or attacks in which there is a loss of consciousness, with a succession of … convulsions."

**Hereditation**: "The influence of heredity."

**Intemperance**: "Excess or lack of self-control in respect to food and drink; immoderate indulgence in the use of alcoholic drinks."

**Leukorrhea**: "A whitish, viscid discharge from the vagina and uterine cavity…. Called also *whites*."

**Lochia**: "The vaginal discharge that takes place during the first week or two after childbirth."

**Marasmus**: "Progressive wasting and emaciation, especially such a wasting in young children when there is no obvious or ascertainable cause."

**Menorrhagia**: "Abnormally profuse menstruation."

**Onanism**: "Masturbation."

**Paralysis**: "A loss of motion or sensation in a living part or member."

**Paroxysm**: "A sudden recurrence or intensification of symptoms."

**Phlegmasia dolens**: "Phlebitis (inflammation of a vein) of the femoral vein, occasionally following parturition (childbirth) and typhoid fever. It is characterized by swelling of the leg, usually without redness."

**Phthisis pulmonalis**: "Pulmonary consumption."[2]

**Prolapsus**: "A protrusion, as well as falling down, of a part of some viscus, so as to be partly external or uncovered."[3]

**Puerperal**: "Pertaining to childbirth"

**Scarlatina**: "Scarlet fever."

---

[1] Definitions for medical terms were obtained from *The American Illustrated Medical Dictionary*, 8th ed. (Philadelphia: W. B. Saunders Co., 1916.)

[2] Joseph Thomas, *A Complete Pronouncing Medical Dictionary…* (Philadelphia, J. B. Lippincott Co., 1889).

[3] *Ibid.*

# Volume 1: 1842–1853

1  **Tilman Barnett**, lunatic from Bibb County, age 30, married, cause and duration of insanity unknown, admitted 15th December 1842, died of maniacal exhaustion 18th June 1843.

2  **George Maxwell**, lunatic (condition demented & cataleptic) convict from the penitentiary age 36, single, cause of insanity confinement in the penitentiary, duration two years, admitted 4th January 1843, escaped slightly improved, Sept 1st 1844, heard from two months afterwards in Savannah.

3  **Moses Harris**, lunatic from Wayne County, age 54, married, cause of insanity, religious excitement, duration unknown, admitted 23rd January 1843, removed by his friends 7th Novr. 1843.

4  **Mrs. Mary Riley**, lunatic from Monroe County, age 47, married, cause of insanity, ungovernable temper, duration unknown, admitted 27th January 1843, discharged cured 16th July 1843, readmitted in a state of furious mania 31st March 1844, died of general paralysis on the 5th March 1847.

5  **Mrs. Catharine G. Latimer**, lunatic from Morgan County, age 32, married, cause of insanity puerperal condition, together with domestic unhappiness, duration unknown, admitted 3rd of June 1843, discharged cured 5th of Oct 1843, re-admitted in a state of violent mania on Sept 18th 1845, from Talbot County, discharged cured 23rd Oct 1848 and immediately afterwards wrote her husband to remove her. Left the institution in company with her husband 3rd Feb 1849. Readmitted on Sept 24 1850.

6  **William Reynolds**, lunatic from the penitentiary, age 20, single, cause and duration of insanity unknown, admitted 8th June 1843, was pardoned by the Governor (his term of servitude not having expired in the penitentiary) and removed by his father (in an improved condition) to North Carolina Oct 9th 1845.

7  **James H. Hall**, lunatic from Greene County, age 23, single, cause and duration unknown, admitted 29th July 1843, discharged cured 20th Sept 1843.

8  **Daniel Ashmore**, lunatic from Liberty County (condition, demented), single, age 30, cause of insanity intense application to study, duration 12 years, admitted 22nd Sept 1843. Found dead in his bed (having been in usual health the day before) on the morning of the 19 December 1847.

9  **Mrs. Joel**, lunatic from Milledgeville, age 94, widow, cause of insanity unknown, duration 30 or 40 years, admitted 4th Oct 1843, died of dysentery & inflammation of intestine, 14th Sept 1845.

"Up to this time persons were supported in the institution by their friends, or by the counties from which they were sent. The legislature at its session of 1843 made a special appropriation of $50 for the support of each pauper that might be sent to the institution. Justices of the Inferior Courts were required to certify to the pauperism of such individuals."

10  **Louisa Ansley**, lunatic from Walton County, pauper, age 24, single, cause of insanity ill health, duration 4 or 5 years, admitted 18[th] January 1844, died Augt 3[rd] 1855.

11  **John Smith**, lunatic from Savannah, pauper, age 49 or 50, single, Irishman & sailor, cause & duration of insanity unknown, admitted 18[th] January 1844, died Octr. 17[th] 1854.

12  **John A. Nelson**, lunatic, pauper from Macon, age 22, clerk in a store, single, cause of insanity an attack of congestive fever, duration six months, admitted 22[nd] January 1844, discharged cured Oct 6, 1844. Visited the institution this day Apr 24[th] 1850, in company with his wife, is now a successful merchant in East Macon, has two children.

13  **Juliana Mayer**, pauper, lunatic & epileptic from Savannah, age 23, single, cause of disease, disappointed affection, duration 4 years, admitted 24[th] January 1844, died of consumption July 31[st] 1853.

14  **Margaret Cavenough**, lunatic, from Savannah, pay patient widow, age 50, cause of disease loss of property, duration 8 or 10 years, admitted 8[th] February 1844, removed by her friends much improved, 26[th] March 1847.

15  **John Wade**, lunatic, pauper from Savannah, age 36, married, engineer and machinist, Englishman, cause of insanity ill health and jealousy, duration two years, admitted 11[th] April 1844, discharged 4[th] July 1844, on promise that he would leave the state. He visited several of the western states, some of the northern states, and finally went to Savannah. They supposed there that he had escaped from the institution. He was immediately arrested and returned to the asylum without any form of commitment August 26[th] 1845. He remained here till the 16[th] December 1845 at which time he made application to the board of trustees for a discharge. They determined that they had no legal right to withhold it and it was granted. When last heard from he was in Charleston at work in a machine shop, still badly insane.

16  **Bridget LaRoux**, lunatic, pauper from Savannah, age 30, married, she would not consent to come to the institution willingly, unless she could be permitted to bring her child (a little boy of two years of age) with her & according to her request the child was sent & the city council of Savh. Paid the asylum at the rates of $50 pr annum for taking care of the child. Cause of insanity abuse from husband, duration 6 months, admitted 17 April 1844, discharged cured 22[nd] December 1844. Was at the asylum in Nov 185[?] seeking employment.

17  **Stephen H. Barton**, lunatic, pauper from Burke County, age 40, married, farmer, cause of insanity intemperance, duration 4 or 5 years, admitted 17[th] February 1844, died of phthysis plumonalis October 31[st] 1855.

18  **Samuel Henderson**, pauper, lunatic, from Cobb County, age 47, married, farmer, cause of disease religious study, duration 10 or 12 years, admitted 23rd March 1844, died March the 12 1855.

19  **Robert Justice**, pauper, lunatic from Laurence [Laurens] County, age 22, married, farmer, cause of insanity intemperance, duration 6 months, admitted 15th April 1844, escaped greatly improved 21st June 1844, entirely recovered soon after getting home, but in the summer of 1845 from habits of intemperance became insane again and was re-admitted under the old commitment July 24th 1845. Eloped entirely sane 29th Sept 1845, would have been discharged in a few days had he remained.

20  **Thos. S. Harrison**, lunatic from Jackson County, pay patient, age 24, single, farmer, cause of insanity, disappointed love, duration 18th months, admitted 26th April 1844, disease hereditary, died 10th Sept 1872.

21  **Nathaniel Mitchell**, pauper, lunatic from Jones County, age 60, single, had lost a leg, cause not known for amputation, cause and duration of insanity unknown, admitted 4th May 1844, removed by his friends 18th May 1844.

22  **Mrs. Temperance Thomas**, lunatic from Jones County, pay patient, age about 40, married, cause & duration of insanity not known, admitted some time in May 1844, brought her servant with her into the institution, removed by her friends 12th July 1844. This patient was not sent here in conformity with the requisitions of the law, but at her own request, in order that she might be near her medical attendant (Dr. Fort). The institution boarded her. She brought her own bedding, servant &c. and was not visited by the res[iden]t phys[icia]n.

23  **William Walton**, monomaniac from Wilkes County, pauper, age 46, married, cause of insanity religious study, duration 10 or 12 years, farmer, admitted 15th May 1844, discharged cured 12th August 1846.

24  **Mathew M. Pinder**, idiot, pauper from Forsyth County, single, age 35, idiocy congenital, admitted June 13th 1844, found dead in his room (having been in usual health the day before) on the morning of the 5th July 1844, post mortem appearances denoted death from apoplexy.

25  **Polly Denning**, pauper, lunatic from Jones County, married, act 50, cause of insanity ill health and jealousy, duration 8 or 10 years, disease hereditary, condition demented, admitted June 15 1844, died 19th Oct 1846 of marasmus, the result of chronic diarrhea.

26  **Solomon Colson**, pauper, lunatic from Wilkinson County, age 36, married, cause of insanity intemperance, duration 1 month, admitted 5th July 1844, discharged on the application of his friends with an order from the Justices of the Inferior Court of the county from which he was sent (unimproved) Aug 17th 1844. Shortly after returning home he entirely recovered, has visited the institution twice since.

27 **Benjamin Hendrick**, pauper, lunatic from Wilkes County, age 60, single, cause of insanity hereditary, duration 15 or 20 years, school teacher, admitted 13th July 1844, had severe ulcers on both legs & was blind, died 8th July 1846 of dysentery and inflammation of his bowels.

28 **Nancy Malone**, alias "British," pauper, lunatic from Pike County, age 65 or 70, single, cause of disease unknown, duration about 30 years, admitted 19th July 1844, died of dysentery and inflammation intestines succeeding measles, 22nd March 1848.

29 **Stephen Harris**, pauper, lunatic and epileptic from Cass County, age 46, married, farmer and miner, cause of disease unknown, duration of epilepsy 15 or 20 years, admitted 23rd July 1844, found dead in his room (having been in usual health the day before) in the morning of the 26th Nov 1847, died in all probability from an attack of apoplexy.

30 **Silas Williams**, pauper, lunatic from Walton County, age 28, married, farmer, cause religious excitement, duration 2 months, admitted August 7th 1844, discharged cured 14 March 1845. When last heard from remained well.

31 **Lucy Branch**, pauper, lunatic from Montgomery County, age 48, married, cause of lunacy ill treatment from her husband and hereditation, duration 6 or 8 years, admitted 19th Aug 1844, died of chronic dysentery 15 July 1847.

32 **LeRoy Paris**, pauper, epileptic from Warren County, age 42, single, cause of epilepsy unknown, duration 12 or 15 years, admitted August 31st 1844, died of congestion of his lungs 29 April 1847.

33 **Elizabeth Harper**, pauper, lunatic from Clarke County, age 50, widow, cause not known, duration 15 years, admitted 7th Sept. 1844, died of atrophy Nov 6th 1845.

34 **Delila Evans**, pauper, idiot from Gwinnett County, age 22, single, idiocy congenital, admitted Sept 28th 1844, died of chronic diarrhea June 5th 1846.

35 **Sophia Young**, pauper, lunatic from Columbia County, age 49, widow, cause of insanity loss of friends, duration 12 or 15 years, admitted Oct 18th 1844, died of consumption May 17th 1852.

36 **Zachariah Hendrick**, pauper, lunatic from Taliaferro County, age 48, single, farmer, cause intemperance, duration 14 years, admitted Oct 24 1844, escaped Feb 3rd 1846 slightly improved, returned July 9th 1846.

37 **Frances Stokes**, pauper, lunatic from Bibb County, age 32, married, cause of disease puerperal, duration 2 months, admitted Oct 28th 1844, discharged cured April 12th 1845.

38 **Joshua Baugh**, pauper, epileptic, from Gwinnett County, age 43, married, farmer, cause of disease not known, duration from infancy, admitted Nov 19th 1844, died of repeated attacks of convulsions 27 Oct 1846.

39  **Nancy Williams**, pauper, lunatic from Pulaski County, married, age 48, cause cessation of catamenia, duration 4 or 5 years, admitted 25th November 1844.

40  **Mrs. Sarah P. Dawson**, pauper, lunatic from Savannah, age 35, married, cause of insanity domestic unhappiness, duration 5 years, admitted November 28th 1844. [R?] by her daughter [Mrs.?] Gibbs, August 1st 186[3?].

41  **Martha C. Johnson**, pauper, lunatic from Monroe County, age 40, widow, cause of derangement domestic trouble, duration 8 years, admitted December 13th 1844, died 21st May 1872.

42  **Mary Scott**, congenital idiot from Cobb County, single, age 23, badly deformed, admitted 6 January 1845, died from exposure whilst travelling to the institution January 7th, 1845.

43  **Tamsey, alias Jane Wheeler**, pauper, idiot from Gwinnett County, age 21, condition rather idiotic though sufficient mind to take care of herself, had an illegitimate child which was sent with her. The Inferior Court of Gwinnett promised to pay $50 per annum for the support of the child. Discharged and sent back to Gwinnett County not considering her a fit subject for the institution 6th Oct 1846.

44  **Sarah Greenwood**, pauper, lunatic from Pulaski County, age 55, married, cause not known, duration 1 year, admitted January 15th 1845, died of dysentery and inflammation of intestines April 2nd 1845.

45  **Nancy Denning**, pauper, lunatic from Jones County, married, age 45, cause hereditation, duration 3 years, admitted 28th Feb 1845, Removed by friends slightly improved, Nov 27th 1845, returned in a much worse condition than when removed, laboring under general paralysis Aug 7th 1847, died April 14th 1851 from an injury of the hand resulting from her breaking the glass in her window.

46  **Caleb Wilkerson**, pauper, lunatic from Troup County, age 49, single, cause of lunacy, disappointed affection, duration 25 or 30 years, common laborer, came of his own accord on foot, without clothing to conceal his nakedness, shoes or hat, had not eaten more than twice or three times while on the road, although he was 5 or 6 days coming. Recd. him Feb 29th 1845, gave him clothing &c., & wrote the Justices of the Inferior Court of his arrival who promised to have him legally committed. They neglected to do so until the 13th May 1846 at which time he was turned out. He then made application in person to the Justices of the Inferior Court of this county for commitment to the asylum which commitment was granted 23rd May 1846 at which time he was recd. as a pauper.

47  **Bryan Smith**, pauper, idiot from Franklin County, age 35, single, idiocy congenital, admitted March 13th 1845, died of marasmus Nov 16th 1845.

48  **Joel H. Dyer**, pauper, lunatic from Franklin County, age 54, married, farmer and shoe maker, became insane while a convict in the penitentiary, duration 3 years, admitted 13th March 1845, died.

49    **John Newman**, pauper, idiot from Campbell County, age 45, single, idiocy congenital, admitted March 16th 1845, died of dysentery 23rd July 1845.

50    **Nancy Shyres**, pauper, lunatic from Franklin County, age 48, single, cause of insanity blow on the head with a hoe from her brother who was in a state of intoxication at the time, duration 15 or 20 years, admitted March 21st 1845, died 4th July 1850 of marasmus.

51    **Mastin Morgan**, pauper, idiot from Madison County, age 14, idiocy congenital, also had epilepsy, admitted 21st March 1845, died of dysentery Nov 5th 1846.

52    **Samuel Harris**, pauper, lunatic from Walton County, age 48, married, blacksmith, cause of insanity bad health, duration 3 years, admitted 25 March 1845, April 1st 1845 escaped, Aug 6th returned by his friends in about the same condition as when he left, removed by his friends 13th Oct 1847, when last heard from remained in a state of derangement. Returned by order of the Inf court of Walton County, April 21st 1849, discharged very greatly improved and went on to recover.

53    **James Washington**, pauper, lunatic from Perry, Houston County, age 72 or 3, widower, sadler and harness maker, cause of disease loss of friends, duration 9 years, admitted 26th March 1845, died of general paralysis 31st July 1848.

54    **Eliza Wilcox**, pauper, lunatic from Muscogee County, age 45, widow, cause and duration of lunacy unknown, admitted 8th May 1845, died of marasmus March 3rd 1854. [additional light writing]

55    **Louisa Robinson**, pauper, lunatic from Stewart County, age 55, widow, cause loss of friends, having lost her husband and children in a short time, duration 3 years, admitted May 10th 1845, died May 17/55.

56    **Moses Woodfin**, pauper, lunatic from Jasper County, age 60, widower, mason and farmer, cause loss of property, duration 12 or 15 years, admitted 15th May 1845, discharged under a promise on his part to go to his sons in Alabama (it not being deemed prudent for him to return to Jasper County) June 7th 1848, returned alone with an application from the Inferior Court of Jasper County for readmittance who promised to commit him soon as the forms of the law could be gone through with, July 9th 1848, very much worsted by his long walk prevations &c., left the asylum without letting any one know where he proposed to go, July 18th 1842, returned along July 24th 1849, discharged 22nd June 1850.

57    **Mrs. Sims**, lunatic from Greensboro, Alabama, pay patient, widow at 50, cause domestic trouble, duration 17 years, admitted June 2nd 1845, discharged cured December 15th 1845.

58    **H. W. Dulin**, pauper, lunatic from Henry County, age 25, single, cause, intemperance, duration 2 years, waggoner, admitted 3rd June 1845, escaped April 17th 1846, when last heard from was at home, still insane,

and indulging in the use of spirits, returned under new commitment Aug 21st 1850 in a state of dementia, died of marasmus July 8th 1852.

59  **Jacob Chadbourne**, pauper, lunatic from Savannah, widower, age 60, formerly merchant, no occupation for several years, admitted 6th June 1845, died 16th Oct 1845 of marasmus.

60  **Hannah Backley**, lunatic from Chatham County, age 45, married, cause cessation of catamenia, duration 1 year, admitted as a pay patient 6th June 1845, transformed to a pauper 20th July 1846, died of dysentery and inflammation of intestines 29th May 1848.

61  **Charity Crews**, epileptic, pauper from Chatham County, age 36, single, cause of epilepsy unknown, duration 31 years, admitted 6th June 1845, died of dysentery 24th Oct 1845.

62  **John James Lenoir**, lunatic from Wilcox County, Alabama, pay patient, age 20, single, student, cause intense application to study, duration 3 years, admitted 11th June 1845, died of anasarea and diarrhea Dec 30th 1851.

63  **Thornton Fitzpatrick**, pauper, lunatic from Forsyth County, married, age 45, farmer and shoemaker, cause of insanity unknown, duration 2 months, admitted 14th June 1845, discharged cured 13st Aug 1846.

64  **John Earle**, pauper, idiot and epileptic from Richmond County, age 22, cause of disease unknown, duration 15 years, admitted 23rd June 1845, died of atrophy Aug 6th 1846.

65  **Polly Hooks**, pauper, lunatic from Putnam County, age 50, widow, cause of disease unknown, duration 15 years, admitted 23rd June 1845, died of inflammation bowels and lungs succeeding measles 16th March 1848.

66  **Harriet Boulevare**, pauper, lunatic and epileptic from Richmond County, age 40, single, cause of disease unknown, duration 15 years, admitted 24th June 1845, died Sept. 2nd 1856.

67  **James James**, pauper, epileptic from Hall County, age 19, single, cause and duration of disease not known, admitted 11th July 1845, died of disease of his heart 27 Feb 1846.

68  **Nancy Blount**, pauper, lunatic from Meriwether County, age 40, married, cause hereditation, duration 3 years (has now a brother in the institution, Capt. Reed), admitted 19th July 1845, discharged cured Oct 17th 1845, readmitted Jany 10th 1854.

69  **Wm. Edward Beddell**, epileptic from Athens, pay patient, age 20, single, student, cause of epilepsy unknown, duration 2 years, admitted 23rd July 1845, found dead in his room (having in all probability died of an attack of apoplexy) on the morning of 5th Nov 1846.

70  **A. Bolivar Seals**, lunatic from Barbour County, Alabama, pay patient, age 19, single, clerk in a dry goods store, cause an attack of congestive

fever, duration 3 months, admitted 4[th] August 1845, discharged cured Oct 6[th] 1845.

71   **Ebenezer Cunningham**, pauper, lunatic from Cobb County, age 37, widower, saddler and harness maker, cause loss of friends, duration 3 months, admitted 15[th] Aug 1845, discharged compos mentis Novr. 25[th] 1845.

72   **Jeremiah Darby**, lunatic from Pike County, Alabama, pay patient, age 37, farmer, married, cause of lunacy ill health and loss of a brother, duration 14[th] months, admitted August 18[th] 1845, escaped (his general health being somewhat improved) 23[rd] Decr. 1845. Returned on foot home, some three months afterwards killed his wife by stabbing her with a long knife in several places about the chest (from an insane motive), was tried for murder in the Superior Court of Montgomery, Alabama, in May 1847 and found "not guilty" upon the plea of insanity. Returned to the asylum May 26[th] 1847. Died of diarrhea September 29[th] 1853.

73   **Spencer Gilbert**, lunatic from Lee County, pauper, age 60, widower, farmer, cause domestic trouble, duration 8 years, admitted Aug 22[nd] 1845, escaped slightly improved Oct 15[th] 1845, returned (in a worse condition than when he left) Nov 15[th] 1845, died 20[th] Oct 1848 of atrophy.

74   **Rebecca Tatum**, pauper, lunatic from Gilmer County, age 30, single, cause disappointed affection, duration 3 years, admitted 30[th] August 1845, died Decr. 28[th] 1854.

75   **Mary McRae**, pay patient, lunatic from Early County, age 40, widow, insanity cause by puerperal convulsions, duration 8 years, admitted Sept 9[th] 1845, died Novr. 1[st] 1862.

76   **Samuel McCraskey**, pauper, lunatic from Habersham County, age 38, single, saddle and harness maker, insanity caused by loss of property and intemperance, duration 8 months, admitted Sept 12[th] 1845, died of concussion of the brain produced by a fall Nov 25[th] 1845.

77   **Jane Paris**, pauper, epileptic from Warren County, age 23-4, single, cause of epilepsy unknown, duration from infancy, admitted 17[th] September 1845, died of continued and repeated attacks of epilepsy, Feb 7[th] 1847.

78   **Keziah Watson**, pauper, lunatic from Laurens County, age 50, married, cause unknown, duration 12 years, admitted Oct 3[rd] 1845, removed by her friends May 2[nd] 1846.

79   **Charlotte Daughtry**, pauper, lunatic from Laurens County, age 35, widow, cause domestic trouble, duration 6 months, admd. Oct 3[rd] 1845, died of dysentery Nov 7[th] 1847.

80   **Mary Craving**, pauper, lunatic from Sumter County, age 50, widow, cause of insanity ill health, was laboring under secondary syphilis at the time of her admission, duration of insanity 6 or 7 years, admitted Oct 5[th] 1845, died of typhoid pneumonia 28[th] March 1846.

81    **Wm. G. Pemble**, pauper, lunatic from Sumter County, age 50, widower, house carpenter and coach maker, cause of disease intemperance, duration 3 months, confined in irons two months of the time, admitted Oct 8[th] 1845, did of apoplexy Oct 16[th] 1845.

82    **Temperance Bracewell**, pauper, epileptic from Laurens County, age 38, single, cause of epilepsy unknown, duration 15 years, admitted 14[th] Oct 1845, died Dec 19, 1850.

83    **Mariah Smith**, pauper, epileptic from Laurens County, age 36, single, has hemiplegia cause not known, duration 5 years, admitted 14[th] Oct 1845, died of typhus fever 18[th] June 1849.

84    **Lewis B. Doane**, lunatic, pay patient from Connecticut, age 25, single, cause of insanity onanism, duration 2 months, admitted 24[th] Oct 1845. This patient left home (Thompson, Con.) in a state of partial insanity, went to New York and there embarked on board the *Celia*, Capt. Thatcher, bound for Savannah. It seems that he was trying to get to his uncles T. B. Haskell of Jones County, Ga. Before the *Celia* reached Savannah he became so furious as to render close confinement necessary. When he reached Sav. he was confined in jail for a short time. He became quiet and was released. He then went to his uncles who soon after brought him to this institution and deposited for his support a small amount of money, stating that his friends at the north were able to pay the necessary amount for his support here. They were written to and after much delay stated that they were unable to pay a dollar. He has been supported upon the charity of the institution ever since. Died July 21, 1854.

85    **Wm. McVinney**, pauper, lunatic from Milledgeville, age 35 or 40, single, seaman, cause and duration of insanity unknown, admitted into the asylum 25[th] Oct 1845, died 20[th] July 1878, marasmus.

86    **James Duncan**, pauper, lunatic from Hancock County, age 45, married, wagon maker, cause of insanity intemperate use of tobacco, spirits, &c., duration 6 or 8 months, admitted 7[th] November 1845, discharged cured March 17[th] 1844, returned home and resumed his ordinary avocation. In a few months however he fell into his old habits of intemperance and relapsed, was returned to the institution in a state of furious mania Dec 2[nd] 1846, died of general paralysis Feb 18[th] 1848.

87    **Jane Tucker**, pauper, lunatic from Stewart County, age 35, married, wife of farmer, admitted Nov 19[th] 1845, died of diarrhea 23[rd] Nov 1846.

88    **John Cole**, pauper, epileptic from Gwinnett County, age 35, married, occupation none, had paralysis of his right arm, admitted 23[rd] Nov 1845, discharged cured April 13[th] 1846, have not heard from him since, epilepsy caused by the intemperate use of spirits, duration 3 years, enlisted in the U.S. service in 1847 and went to Mexico.

89 **Elizabeth Featherstone**, lunatic from Putnam County, pay patient, single, age 60, cause of insanity unknown, duration 15 or 20 years, admitted 28th Nov 1845.

90 **Samuel Sweat**, pauper, lunatic from Ware County, age 40, married, farmer, cause of insanity jealousy, duration 2 years, admitted 19th December 1845, escaped unimproved July 7th 1846, when last heard from was still insane, confined closely at home.

91 **Russell Stowers**, pauper, lunatic from Gwinnett County, single, age 45, common laborer, cause of insanity unknown, duration six months, admitted in the last stage of phthisis pulmonalis, on the 22nd December 1845, died of the same disease 7th January 1846.

92 **James Killingsworth**, pauper, idiot from Gwinnett County, age 45, single, occupation none, condition congenital, admitted January 2nd 1846, died of atrophy 17th December 1846.

93 **Whitson Rosseau**, pauper, lunatic from Putnam County, age 24, single, common laborer, cause unknown, perhaps "onanism", duration 4 years, admitted 9th January 1846, died Sept. 14th 1854.

94 **Jasper Favor**, pauper, epileptic from Putnam County, age 20, single, cause of epilepsy, injury of his head, duration 4 years, died of general paralysis 30th April 1848.

95 **Atha Waters**, pauper, idiot and epileptic child from Paulding County, age 5, admitted January 10th 1846, died in convulsions 27th May 1848.

96 **Richard M. Williams**, lunatic from Savannah, pay patient, age 37, single, cause of lunacy religious enthusiasm, duration 10 or 12 years, admitted January 19th 1846, died 11th Oct 1877, convulsions, no one to notify.

97 **Elizabeth McLendon**, pauper, lunatic from Appling County, age 75 or 80, married cause of disease unknown, duration 25 or 30 years, admitted 19th January 1846, died of dysentery 28th May 1846.

98 **Mary Lee**, pauper, lunatic from Newton County, age 34, widow, cause of disease unknown, duration 7 or 8 years, was attacked with semicrania soon after the inception of her insanity which produced total blindness in one eye, admitted 21st January 1846, died of marasmus complicated with diarrhea on the 29th of September 1849.

99 **Judah Delt**, congenital pauper, idiot and deformed from Lee County, age 13, very small and much emaciated, admitted 3rd Feb 1846, died of marasmus April 5th 1847.

100 **James Delt**, congenital pauper, idiot, deformed and blind from Lee County, age 7, admitted 3rd February 1846, died of dysentery 19th May 1846.

101 **Andrew Perfue** (Pole), pauper, lunatic from Bibb County, age 55 or 60, cause and duration of disease not known, admitted 5th Feb 1846, died of phthisis pulmonalis 16th April 1849.

102 **Calvin Majors**, pauper, lunatic from Carroll County, age 24, single, farmer, cause of lunacy religious study, duration 4 years, admitted 17th Feb 1846, died of chronic diarrhea June 6th 1851.

103 **Mary Jane O'Neall**, pauper, lunatic from Tattnall County, age 25 or 6, single, cause of disease religious study, duration 2 years, admitted 10th March 1846, died of inflammation of intestines June 22nd 1849.

104 **William Fletcher**, pauper, lunatic from Henry County, age 37, single, common laborer, cause of insanity intemperate use of spirits and tobacco, duration three years, admitted May 6th 1846, escaped Aug 27th 1849, returned Oct 22nd 1847, escaped Nov 3rd 1851, returned voluntarily Dec 3rd 1850. Died 20 Jan 1898, old age.

105 **Ann B. Walker**, lunatic from Richmond County, age 47, widow, insanity caused by loss of friends and an inveterate cutaneous eruption, duration 10 or 12 years, admitted 10th June 1846, died July 27th 1856.

106 **Caroline M. McMillan**, lunatic from Quincy, Florida, pay patient, age 41, married, cause of insanity cessation of catamenia, duration 8 months, admitted 17th June 1846, discharged, cured 20th May 1847.

107 **Redick P. Hammock**, pauper, lunatic from Laurens County, age 40, married, house carpenter, cause of disease intemperance, duration 3 or 4 years, admitted 17th June 1846, died 17th Nov 1846 from the formation of several enormously large sloughing ulcers on various parts of his body, but principally along his spine.

108 **Nicholas Tuttle** (Irishman), pauper, lunatic from Savannah, age 38, single, wagoner, cause of disease disappointed affection, duration 3 months, admitted 20th June 1846, died Jan 12th 1851 of inflammation of the abdomen.

109 **Anderson Quick**, pauper, lunatic from Fayette County, age 26, single, laborer, insanity caused by solitary confinement, duration 8 years, was chained to one spot during the whole period, admitted 28th June 1846, died of marasmus 11th May 1847.

110 **Sarah A. E. F. Hines**, lunatic from Macon, pay patient, single, age 38 or 9, cause of insanity ill health, duration 2 years, admitted 7th July 1846, removed greatly improved 21st Nov. 1848, carried to the asylum in Columbia S.C. in June 1850.

111 **Margaret A. B. Harvey**, lunatic from Mareanna, Florida, age 37, single, pay patient, cause of insanity not known, duration 8 or 10 years, admitted July 11th 1846, died 3rd Aug 1877, marasmus, sister notified by Dr. Powell.

112 **Redmund Hutchins**, pauper, lunatic from Cobb County, age 65, married, farmer, insanity caused by religious study, duration 3 years, admitted 28th July 1846, removed by his friends an unimproved 15th Oct 1847.

113 **Polly Ann Brown**, pauper, lunatic from Henry County, age 45, single, insanity has existed from early life, no cause known, admitted 20th August 1846, died of dysentery 25th Sept 1847.

114 **William Henry Lewis**, pauper, lunatic from LaGrange, Troup County, age 45, single, insanity caused by intemperance, duration 15 years, admitted 20th Aug. 1846.

115 **Elvira Hurt**, pauper, lunatic from Cass County, age 45, married, cause and duration of insanity not known, admitted 21st Aug. 1846, found dead in her room on the morning of the 30th Sept. 1846, having in all probability died of some disease of the heart.

116 **Jacob L. Abrahams**, lunatic from Coweta County, age 47, married, farmer, formerly merchant, pay patient, insanity caused by domestic trouble and loss of property, duration 12 or 15 years, escaped Nov 7th 1846, returned by his friends Nov 28th 1847, escaped again on 15th March 1848, when last heard from was at home, attending to his ordinary business, though still badly insane.

117 **Harvey R. Kemp**, pauper, lunatic from Forsyth County, age 23, married, farmer, cause of insanity unknown, duration 10 months, admitted 30th Aug 1846, removed by his friends May 9th 1847, died at home sometime in July 1849.

118 **Mary Whitlock**, pauper, lunatic from Forsyth County, age 47, married, cause of disease "ill treatment by her husband", duration 5 or 6 years, admitted 30th Aug 1846, died of phthisis pulmonalis Sept 15th 1848.

119 **Joshu[a] Johnson**, congenital, partial pauper, idiot from Cobb County, admitted 29th Sept 1846, died of bronchitis 29th February 1848.

120 **Wiley Cummings**, pauper, lunatic from Telfair County, age 30, married, farmer, cause of insanity jealousy (well founded), duration one month, admitted 28th Oct 1846, discharged cured 2nd June 1847.

121 **Elizabeth P. Morrison**, lunatic from Glenville, Barbour County, Alabama, pay patient, age 60, married, cause of disease ill health, duration 10 or 12 years, admitted 6th Nov 1846, died July 22nd 1851.

122 **Robert Moss**, pauper, lunatic from DeKalb County, age 18, single, laborer, cause of condition not known, duration 1 year, admitted Nov 7th 1846, removed by his father 27th Sept 1848, returned May 5th 1849, Died Septr. 29th 1854.

123 **Benjn. J. Harper**, lunatic from Hancock County, pay patient, age 21, single, farmer, cause of disease intemperance, duration 3 months, admitted 19th Nov 1846, discharged cured Feb 19th 1846.

124 **Martha Wallace**, pauper, lunatic from Morgan County, age 50, widow, cause of derangement not known, duration 10 or 12 years, admitted 20th Nov 1846, died July 15th 1851.

125 **Mary Waller**, pauper, lunatic and epileptic from Cobb County, age 40, widow, cause of condition not known, duration 4 or 5 years, admitted 23rd Nov 1846, died of exhaustion from epilepsy August 5th 1853.

126 **Harriet Gadis**, congenital pauper, idiot from Cherokee County, age 18, admitted 8th December 1846, died 30 Dec 1909, pneumonia, buried here.

127 **William Gadis**, congenital pauper, idiot from Cherokee County, age 16, admitted 8th December 1846.

128 **William Pool**, pauper, epileptic from Baker County, age 40, widower, farmer, cause and duration of epilepsy unknown, admitted 31st December 1846, found dead in his room on the morning of the 17th March 1847, having died (as supposed) from an attack of apoplexy.

129 **Doct Oliver P. Kelton**, lunatic from Galveston, Texas, age 35, married, cause, domestic trouble and intemperance, duration 15 days, admitted 15th Jan 1847, discharged cured and employed by the Trustees as an attendant at the institution on the 5 July 1847, went to Milledgeville, got into a state of intoxication and left, said he was going to Texas 14th July 1847, returned by Major Pope of Clinton in a state of perfectly furious mania on the 17th July 1847, received him and permitted him to remain at pleasure, on the 22 August 1847 he again left the asylum without informing any one of his intentions, heard nothing from him till Nov 5th 1847 at which time he returned of his own accord, quite rational and asked permission to stop for a while, it was granted and he remained until the 24th January 1848 at which time he again left, said he was going up the country to teach school, returned to the asylum 14 July 1849, has been rambling in Georgia, Tennessee, Kentucky, Ohio &c, has drank some and a part of the time was deranged, is perhaps partially insane now, became very troublesome in the neighborhood, was arrested and committed to the Milledgeville jail as a lunatic Aug 27 1849, brought out to the Asylum to await his trial 2nd Sept 1849, court convened and failed to convict him, he then came out got his clothing and left without stating where he proposed to go Sept 13 1849.

130 **Bethia Wright**, pauper, lunatic from Lumpkin County, age 24, married, cause, "abuse from husband," duration 5 years, admitted 15th January 1847.

131 **Nathaniel R. Hood**, pauper, epileptic from Franklin County, age 47, married, farmer, formerly merchant, cause, intemperance, duration 5 years, admitted 17th January 1847, removed by friends Aug 10th 1848, returned by his friends Oct 22 1850 without commitment with the requisition that he shall be regularly recommitted within twenty days, has not been recommitted and discharged June 10th 1851.

132 **Sarah Comstock** (Irish woman), pauper, lunatic from Savannah, age 20, married, cause "abuse from husband," duration 1 year, admitted 26 Jan 1847, died 7 Oct 1875, congestive chill.

133 **Carlisle Coleman**, congenital, deformed pauper, idiot, from Cobb County, age 25, admitted 31$^{st}$ January 1847, died suddenly 9$^{th}$ Feb 1847, cause of his death not known.

134 **Jemima Oliver**, pauper lunatic from Cobb County, single, age 30, cause disappointed affection, duration 3 years, admitted 31$^{st}$ January 1847, died of mirasmus June 4$^{th}$ 1852.

135 **William Lewis** (Englishman), pauper lunatic from Cass County, age 22, single, clerk, cause intemperance, duration one month, admitted 3$^{rd}$ Feb 1847, discharged cured Aug 20$^{th}$ 1847.

136 **John Talmadge**, lunatic from Athens, pay patient, age 55, married, mechanic, cause jealousy and intemperance, duration 6 or 7 years, admitted 19$^{th}$ Feb 1847, discharged 30$^{th}$ Oct 1847. This patient spent a few months in this institution in 1843, but no account can be found of his admission or discharge. He was discharged at that time as cured. Died June 1849 at home of dysentery.

137 **"Minte"**, a pauper lunatic girl from Pike County, age 15, single, cause and duration of insanity unknown, admitted 3$^{rd}$ March 1847, discharged 23$^{rd}$ Oct 1848. As there has been no opportunity of sending her home she is yet in the institution Feb 1$^{st}$ 1849. Do. [Ditto] Oct 2$^{nd}$ 1849. Still in the institution Oct 9$^{th}$ 1850. Left the institution for Griffin Feb 26 1851.

138 **Penelope Saunders**, idiot from Vineville, paypatient, age 18, idiocy congenital, admitted 16$^{th}$ April 1847, died Febry 18$^{th}$ 1852.

139 **Benjn. Mason**, lunatic from Jones County, age 45, pay patient, married, overseer, cause intense application to study in an attempt to write a work on agriculture, duration 2 weeks, admitted 24$^{th}$ April 1847, removed by his friends greatly improved 1$^{st}$ Sept 1847. When last heard from was not entirely well, but had sufficiently recovered to enable him to prosecute his ordinary business of life. Subsequently recovered after which visited and spent a night at the asylum.

140 **John Bradley**, partial idiot and lunatic from Macon, pay patient, age 20, single, occupation none, cause unknown, duration from early life, admitted 26$^{th}$ April 1847.

141 **George Frederick Houser**, pauper lunatic from Augusta, age 30, married, engineer and machinist, cause intemperance, duration 2 or 3 months, adm. 29$^{th}$ April 1847, discharged cured 6$^{th}$ Sept 1847.

142 **Majr. Isaiah Attaway**, lunatic from Twiggs County, age 45, married, farmer and mechanic, cause hereditation, duration 9 or 10 years, admitted 11$^{th}$ May 1847, removed by his wife 10$^{th}$ Sept 1847, returned Oct 6$^{th}$ 1847, discharged on account of his friends failing to supply the necessary amt. of money for his support in the institution, January 23$^{rd}$ 1848.

143 **Mary Ann Allen**, lunatic from Upson County, age 40, married, pay patient, cause [blank], duration [blank], admitted 21$^{st}$ May 1847, removed

3rd May 1877, improved. Returned 30th March 1878. Address 1884 Sarah Adams, Augusta Ga., Sarah Walker, [illegible on film], Florida.

144 **Littleton G. Adams**, pauper epileptic from Henry County, age 26, farmer, married, cause not known, duration 2 years, admitted 1st June 1847, died of congestion of his brain 15th March 1848.

145 **Henry Johnson**, pauper epileptic from Lee County, age 60, single, laborer, cause and duration unknown, admitted 6th June 1847, discharged 23rd Oct 1848 as well not having had a convulsion, since his admission was permitted however at his own request till the 16th January 1849, at which time he died of congestion of his brain.

146 **William S. Bower**, pauper lunatic from Milledgeville, age 29, single, laborer, cause unknown, duration 6 or 7 years, admitted 5th July 1847, died of inflammation of the intestines May 17th 1851.

147 **Charles Farell**, pauper lunatic from Forsyth County, age 60, married, farmer and school teacher, cause hereditation, duration 2 years, admitted 15th August 1847, discharged sufficiently restored to be returned home and pursue his ordinary business, when last heard from was entirely well, ~~Sept 24th 1848~~ Nov 3rd 1848 1849 March 25, Is entirely sane and attends to his business punctually.

148 **William J. D. Smiley**, lunatic from Crawford County, pay patient, age 30, single, school teacher, cause disappointed love, duration 3 years, admitted 20th August 1847, escaped unimproved Oct 2nd 1847, returned much worse under new commitment 27 March 1850, escaped July 2nd 1850.

149 **Emily Kirkpatrick**, lunatic from Monticello, pay patient, age 24, married, cause ill health, duration 6 months, admitted 22 Sept 1847, died Jan [or June] 1st 1858.

150 **Sarah Pickens**, congenital idiot, pauper from Madison County, age 23, single, admitted 24th Sept 1847, died of dysentery 26th March 1848.

151 **Adeline Smith**, pauper lunatic and epileptic from Campbell County, age 15, single, cause sudden healing of a large abscess that had been discharging matter for a great while, duration 8 or 10 years, admitted Oct 5th 1847, died of atrophy 25th December 1847.

152 **Benjamin F. Askew**, lunatic from Hancock County, pay patient, age 24, single, farmer, cause intemperance, duration 3 months, admitted 20th Oct 1848, discharged cured 12th January 1848.

153 **Mary Ann Usher**, pauper lunatic from Cobb County, age 30, married, cause unknown, duration 3 or 4 years, admitted Oct 26th 1847, died of phthisis pulmonalis 10th Sept 1849.

154 **Frances McElhannon**, pauper lunatic and epileptic from Paulding County, age 13, cause injury of her head, duration 11 years, admitted 5th Nov 1847, died June 11th 1855.

155  **Morgan Dean**, congenital pauper idiot from Paulding County, age 26, single, admitted 5[th] Nov 1847, died of inanition Aug 26[th] 1851.

156  **Susannah Dean**, pauper idiot from Paulding County, age 18, condition congenital, admitted 5[th] Nov 1847, died of typhoid pneumonia succeeding measles, 6[th] March 1848.

157  **Lafayette Dean**, congenital pauper idiot from Paulding County, age 8, admitted 5[th] Nov 1847, died of atrophy Nov 18[th] 1851.

158  **Henry G. Mathews**, lunatic from Columbus, age 23, single, tailor, cause hereditation and ill health, duration 12 months, admitted 10[th] Nov 1847, discharged cured 21[st] Oct 1848, returned home and some time in November following was attacked with epileptiform convultions which continued till some time in Apr. 1849 at which time he died.

159  **Frederick Campbell**, lunatic from Camden, Wilcox County, pay patient, age 60, married, farmer and merchant, cause hereditation, duration [blank], admitted 26[th] Nov 1847, died of chronic diarrhea supposed to have been produced by ulceration of his intestines, 12[th] February 1848.

160  **Dr. James McWhorter**, pauper lunatic from Carroll County, age 28, single, cause intemperance, duration 1 year, admitted 27[th] November 1847, escaped 6[th] Decr. 1847, when last heard from was at home, returned under new commitment Dec 19[th] 1851, badly deranged, died ~~Dec~~ Novr. 15[th] 1854.

161  **Solomon Mabry**, pauper lunatic from Troup County, age 42, married, farmer, cause and duration of lunacy unknown (recent), admitted 29[th] Nov 1847, discharged cured 7[th] June 1848.

162  **Jeremiah Touchstone**, pauper lunatic and epileptic from Lowndes County, age 21, single, laborer, cause of disease unknown, duration 11 years, admitted 7 Decr 1847, died of chronic diarrhea 28 Feb 1850.

163  **John Dalrymple**, congenital deformed pauper idiot from Lumpkin County, age 43, admitted 17[th] Decr. 1847, found dead in his room on the morning of the 29[th] Decr. 1847, no cause known.

164  **Hiram N. Wilson**, pauper lunatic from Augusta, age 46, married, "stage contractor," cause intemperance, duration ~~12 months~~ unknown, admitted 17[th] Decr. 1847, died of chronic diarrhea succeeding dysentery June 10[th] 1849.

165  **Joseph Hall**, pauper lunatic from Gwinnett County, age 35, single, farmer, admitted 21[st] December 1847, cause religious study, duration 2 months, escaped from institution May 23[rd] 1852, returned May 30[th] 1852 of his own accord.

166  **Doct. Sterling F. Edmunds**, pauper lunatic from Columbus, age 43, married, admitted 29[th] December 1847, cause intemperance, duration three months, died of ulceration of the intestines 21[st] Oct 1848.

167 **Martin Costelow** (Irishman), pauper lunatic from Muscogee County, age 44, married, farmer, cause unknown, duration ~~three months~~, admitted 29[th] December 1847, [blank] Augt. 9[th] 1854.

168 **Josiah H. Reed**, pauper lunatic from Muscogee County, age 47, single, laborer, cause hereditation, duration 15 or 20 years, admitted 29[th] December 1847, died of general dropsy March 31, 1850.

169 **Henry W. Head**, pauper lunatic from Fayette County, age 31, married, farmer, cause unknown, duration 4 years, admitted 6[th] Jany 1848, died 14[th] April 1869.

170 **Richard J. Milner**, pauper lunatic from Fayette County, age 40, single, school teacher, cause hereditation and disappointed affection, duration 2 years, admitted 6[th] Jan 1848, escaped July 10[th] 1850, returned July 11[th] 1850, escaped Aug 1[st] 1851, returned Aug 4[th], died Mar 21[st] 1861.

171 **Jessee Miller**, pauper epileptic from Jefferson County, age 25, single, laborer, cause unknown, duration 11 years, admitted 12[th] January 1848, died of typhoid fever on 7[th] August 1849.

172 **James McLanahan**, pauper lunatic from Walker County, age 40, married shoe maker, cause intemperance, duration 2 years, admitted 14[th] January 1848, discharged "compass mentis" Oct 23[rd] 1848, left the institution for home January 25[th] 1849.

173 **Riley Pearce**, pauper idiot from Houston County, age 21, congenital idiocy, admitted 19[th] Feb 1848, died of atrophy 14[th] Sept 1849.

174 **Maranda Pearce**, pauper idiot from Houston County, age 23, condition congenital, admitted 19[th] Feb 1848, died of marasmus 25 Aug 1849.

175 **Lavicy Webb**, pauper lunatic from Troup County, age 35, married, cause domestic trouble and ill health, duration 8 years, admitted 19[th] Feb 1848, died of consumption November 5[th] 1852.

176 **Alexander McRanie**, pauper epileptic and paralytic from Telfair County, age 23, single, cause not known, duration from childhood, admitted 3[rd] March 1848, died in convulsions May 9[th] 1849.

177 **Silas Brown**, pauper lunatic from Fayette County, age 36, shoe maker, married, cause and duration of disease not known, has but one leg, admitted 24[th] March 1848, died of typhoid fever Aug 7[th] 1849.

178 **Elizabeth Huff**, lunatic from Walker County, age 40, married, pay patient, cause domestic trouble, ill health and the immoderate use of tobacco, duration 7 or 8 years, admitted 13[th] April 1848, removed improved 26[th] April 1877, address P. W. Strozier, Greenville, Geo.

179 **Lavina Clarke**, pauper lunatic from Early County, age 44, widow, cause not known, duration 6 years, admitted 15 April 1848, died of consumption September 13[th] 1853.

180 **Rebecca Goodson**, pauper lunatic from Bryan County, age 39, widow, cause domestic troubles, duration 7 years, admitted 23rd April 1848, died of thisis pulmonalis July 20 1859.

181 **John Bird**, pauper lunatic from Warren County, age 40, single, laborer, cause and duration of disease not known, admitted 3rd May 1848, died June 10th 1861.

182 **James O'Brien**, lunatic from Milledgeville, pay patient, age 60, cause intemperance, duration 1 year, married, grocer, admitted 8th May 1848, removed by his friends April 16th 1849.

183 **Peter Leddy**, pauper lunatic from Jones County, age 35, single, tailor, cause not known, duration 2 weeks, admitted 10th May 1848, discharged cured 20th Oct 1848, relapsed and recommitted, received at the asylum June 9th 1851, duration of insanity a few months.

184 **Benjamin Hodges**, lunatic from Bulloch County, pay patient, age 45, single, cause not known, duration 12 years, farmer, admitted 17th May 1848, escaped 31st May 1848.

185 **John W. Lee**, lunatic from Clarke County, pay patient, age 35, single, farmer, cause "onanism" or failure in business or both, duration 2 or 3 years, admitted 31 May 1848, died of chronic irritation in the intestines probably deep, ulcerations did exist, June 19th 1851.

186 **James D. Atkinson**, lunatic from Savannah, age 29, single, pauper, cause disappointed affection and want of employment, duration 1 month, admitted 2nd June 1848, discharged cured Jan 16th 1849.

187 **Col. Peter F. Mahone**, lunatic from Talbotton, pay patient, age 50, married, hotel keeper, cause intemperance, duration 5 years, admitted 8th June 1848, discharged as sufficiently restored to return to his home, Aug 10th 1849.

188 **James King**, pauper lunatic from Ware County, age 35, married, farmer, cause not known, duration 5 months, admitted 4th July 1848, died Octr. 4th 1854.

189 **Thos. McBee**, pauper, epileptic from Walker County, age 30, married, farmer, cause ill health, duration 2 years, admitted 7th July 1848, discharged as sufficiently restored to make such a course proper, July 2nd 1849.

190 **Ann B. Pearce**, pauper lunatic from Decatur County, age 49 or 50, widow, cause not known, duration 8 or 10 years, admitted 28th July 1848.

191 **Preston Hampton**, pauper lunatic from Lumpkin County, age 40, married, farmer, cause religious, duration 3 or 4 months, admitted 3rd Aug 1848, discharged cured 23rd Oct 1848, started for home 6th Decr. 1848.

192 **Margaret Black**, pauper lunatic from Troup County, age 48, married, wife of preacher, cause ill health and domestic trouble, duration 2 months,

admitted 8[th] August 1848, discharge cured August 15[th] 1849, readmitted Nov 29[th] 1850 as a pay patient, discharged Oct 1[st] 1852 but still remains in this institution Jan 1[st] 1852, died 28[th] Feby. 1872, dropsy.

193 **Peterson Black**, lunatic from Troup County, pay patient, age 42, married, preacher, husband of the above patient, duration 2 or 3 weeks, cause the insanity of his wife, admitted 2[nd] Sept. 1848, died of ulceration of his intestines July 29[th] 1849.

194 **John B. Milner**, pauper lunatic from Monroe County, age 38, married, laborer, cause ill health, duration several years, admitted 15 Sept 1848, died Apl 18[th] 1855.

195 **Thos. Lee**, lunatic from Bulloch County, pay patient, age 23, single, laborer, cause masturbation, duration 6 years, admitted 19[th] Sept 1848, removed by his friends 27[th] December 1848, died some time in the summer of 1849 at home.

196 **Patsey Warren**, pauper lunatic from Hall County, age 24, single, cause and duration of disease not known (recent), admitted 23[rd] Sept 1848, disharched Oct 22[nd] 1849, cured.

197 **Sarah Dyke**, lunatic from Tallahassee, Florida, pay patient, age 24, married, cause ill health and religious excitement, duration 1 month, admitted 11[th] Oct 1848, died 12[th] November 1875, paralysis, notified by Dr. Green.

198 **Sarah Cliett**, partial idiot from Macon County, Alabama, pay patient, age 10, cause congestive fever, duration 8 or 9 years, admitted Oct 22[nd] 1848, died 28 Oct 1904, apoplexy. 1892 Sept 17 Mr. T. S. Cliett, Shorter, Macon County, Ala. 10-16-92, Mr. T. C. Cliett, Patterson, Walker Co. Tex., her father.

199 **John K. Snelson**, pauper lunatic from Wilkes County, age 24, single, laborer, cause not known, duration 6 or 7 weeks, admitted Oct 23[rd] 1848, discharged cured Sept 4[th] 1850, readmitted Sept 17[th] 1850, escaped from the asylum Feb 8[th] 1851.

200 **Eliza Neely**, pauper lunatic from Hall County, age 38, widow, cause, ill health and loss of property, duration 6 or 7 years, admitted Nov 2[nd] 1848, discharged Oct 1[st] 1857, discharged 23[rd] July 1872.

201 **Susannah Walden**, pauper lunatic and epileptic from Montgomery County, age 28, widow, cause unknown, duration 20 years, admitted 23[rd] Nov 1848, died of "typhoid affection" 21[st] January 1849.

202 **Isaac Rowdon**, lunatic from Talladega County, Alabama, pay patient, age 55, married, farmer, cause religious study, duration 26 years, admitted 7[th] December 1848, died 23[rd] July 1873.

203 **Martha Mound**, pauper lunatic and epileptic from Screven County, age 22, single, cause unknown, duration 8 or 10 years, admitted 8[th] Decr 1848, died from dystentery Sept 26 1854.

204 **Patrick Hurley** (Irish), pauper lunatic from Butts County, age 40, single, well digger and ditcher, cause intemperance, duration 6 months, admitted 19th Decr 1848, discharged Octr 13 1855.

205 **Lydia Ann Smith**, lunatic from Eufaula, Alabama, pay patient, age 42, married, cause ill health and domestic trouble, duration 10 years, admitted 18th January 1849, discharged 12th Nov 1866.

206 **Emily Brown**, pauper idiot from Gwinnett County, age 24, single, cause unknown, duration 18 or 20 years, admitted 3rd Feb 1849, died 20th Oct 1855.

207 **Sarah Spruce**, pauper lunatic from Floyd County, age 43, widow, cause not known, duration 16 years, admitted Feb 27, 1849, discharged Oct 13, 1853.

208 **James Sinn**, lunatic from Cass County, pay patient, single, age 25 or 6, laborer, cause "disappointed affection," duration 5 years, admitted March 1st 1849, discharged Oct 22nd 1849, readmitted in slightly worse condition Dec 21 1850.

~~209 **John J. Holmes**, pay patient, lunatic and paralytic from Washington Co, age 40, farmer, married, cause apoplexy, duration 5 or 7 years, admitted March 30th 1847.~~

209 **John H. Varnum**, pauper lunatic from Jackson County, age 24, single, farmer, cause suppressed perspiration or "Miller[illegible]," or fright from the death of a gentleman with whom he was sleeping and the consequent suspicions upon the minds of some that he was in some way accessory to his death, duration 4 years, admitted March 31st 1849, died of chronic diarrhea and general debility, June 7th 1851.

210 **William T. Tylor**, pauper epileptic from Pike County, single, laborer, age 24, cause hereditation, duration 6 years, admitted 31st March 1849.

211 **Rachel Kenney**, pauper idiot from Gwinnett County, age 40 or 45, single, condition congenital, admitted April 5th 1849, died of marasmus Apr 22nd 1849.

212 **John D. Holmes**, pauper lunatic from Washington County, age 40, farmer, married, cause apoplexy, duration 6 or 7 years, admitted 6th April 1849, died of dysentery Sept 28th 1850.

213 **Mary Howard**, pauper lunatic from Pike County, age 52, widow, cause ill health and hanging of husband, duration 3 years, admitted 7th April 1849, removed by her brother March 25th 1851.

214 **Miss Delila Porter**, pay patient, lunatic from Calhoun County (Blountstown), Florida, single, age 35, cause ill health, duration 10 years, but more particularly for the last 5 years, admitted 14th April 1849, discharge of May 15 1857.

215 **Ezekiel Clark**, pauper lunatic from Columbus, single, age and occupation unknown, cause and duration of disease unknown, admitted 14th April 1849, discharged cured Dec 1st 1849, readmitted Nov 15th 1850, escaped much improved April 23 1851.

216 **David Fox**, pauper lunatic from DeKalb County, age about 50, social condition, occupation and cause of disease unknown, duration 4 years, maniacal for 3 months, admitted 27th April 1849, died of atrophy Dec 16th 1849.

217 **John H. Casteel**, pauper epileptic from Union County, age 28, single, laborer, cause not known, duration 10 years, admitted 30th April 1849, died suddenly of apoplexy July 1st 1849.

218 **Jeptha J. Hammock**, a pauper lunatic from Jasper County, age 32, married, farmer, cause hereditation, duration 5 weeks, admitted 5 May 1849, discharged cured 16th Sept 1849.

219 **Wm. Moss**, pauper lunatic from DeKalb County, age 46, married, cause not known, duration of present attack two months, had a previous one which lasted for 12 or 14 months, admitted 5th May 1849, discharged cured August 1st 1849, readmitted Jany 12 1854, discharged May 15th 1854.

220 **Mrs. Lavina Green**, pauper lunatic from Houston County, age 38 or 40, married, cause and duration of disease unknown, admitted 13th May 1849, discharged cured May 1st 1850, employed as a regular attendant in the asylum Decr 30th 1850 and doing well.

221 **Willis Tylor**, pauper epileptic from Pike County, age 44, married, laborer, cause not known, duration 15 or 20 years, admitted May 14th 1849, died of paralysis March 9th 1853.

222 **Mrs. Mariah F. Osborne**, lunatic pay patient from Macon, age about 70, married, cause hereditation, duration 25 or 30 years, admitted 19th May 1849, discharged Oct 22nd 1849, but remained for some time.

223 **Joel A. Crane**, pauper lunatic from Cherokee County, age 35 or 6, married farmer, cause injury of his head, duration 4 months, admitted 30th June 1849, died Oct 1st 1849.

224 **Mrs. Alice Lamb**, pauper lunatic from Randolph County, age 37 or 8, married, wife of farmer, cause "ungovernable disposition and loss of child," duration 7 or 8 years, admitted 8th July 1849.

225 **Lucinda Carr**, pauper lunatic from Bibb County, age 8, single, insane for 4 years, cause congestion of brain during an attack of scarlatina, admitted 30th July 1849, removed by her friends on the 20 Dec 1851 and on 26th of March 1851 had not been returned and was deducted from the number of patients in the asylum at that time.

226 **Dennis Ashford**, a pauper lunatic and epileptic from Richmond County, age 45, married, cause not known, duration 11 years, admitted 3 August 1849, escaped from the institution Aug 16th 1851, readmitted June 10th 1852

in a worse condition than when he eloped from the asylum, eloped May 29 1858, returned May 1/54.

227 **James Garigan Jr.**, a congenital pauper idiot and epileptic from Richmond County, age 14, admitted 3rd August 1849, died Oct 11th 1851.

228 **William Knight** (Englishman), pauper lunatic from Columbus, age 40, married, sailor, cause well founded jealousy, duration six months, admitted 15 August 1849, discharged restored, Decr 18th 1849.

229 **Moses Rolm** (German), lunatic from Montgomery, Alabama, age 24, single, tailor, cause of insanity unknown, duration 1 year, admitted 18th August 1849, removed by his brother and taken to Germany April 16, 1859.

230 **John W. Davis**, pauper lunatic from DeKalb County, age 18, single, farmer, cause of disease not known, duration 6 months, admitted 21st Aug 1849, died of consumption Oct 4th 1855.

231 **James P. Heidt**, pauper lunatic from Savannah, age 16, single, student, cause of disease not known, perhaps religious excitement, duration 7 weeks, admitted 22 Aug 1849, discharged restored Feb 26th 1850.

232 **Caroline Edwards, alias Edmonds, alias McS[cut off]**, pauper lunatic from Gilmer County, age about 48, cause duration, social condition all not known, admitted on the 20th Sept 1849, gave birth to a healthy living male child March 6th 1850, died 25th Jany 1869.

233 **Frederick Turberville**, pauper epileptic from Houston County, age 19, cause not known, duration from infancy, single, admitted 23 Sept 1849, died comatose March 6th 1851.

234 **John R. Manson**, lunatic from Henry County, pay patient, age 21 or 2, single, clerk in a dry goods tore, cause not known, believed masturbation, duration [blank], admitted 29 Sept 1849, died 22 Sept 1908, lobar pneumonia, buried here.

235 **Martha B. Teat**, pauper lunatic from Putnam County, age 42, social condition cause and duration of disease not known, admitted 30th Sept 1849, discharged cured 2nd Sept 1850.

236 **Wm. Miller**, pauper lunatic from Butts County, age about 70, widower, cause and duration of insanity not known, admitted Oct 18th 1849, died of atrophy 18th April 1850.

237 **Jackson Milner**, a pauper lunatic from Henry County, age 32, single, farmer, cause of insanity hereditation, duration 8 months, general health pretty good, admitted Oct 19th 1849, escaped from the asylum Dec 30th 1849, readmitted January 16th 1856. Died.

238 **Mrs. Mary Whit**, lunatic pay patient from Talbot County, age about 35, widow, cause of insanity disordered health, duration two years or more, general health apparently pretty good at this time, admitted Oct 25th 1849, escaped from the institution February 7th 18[cut off in binding].

239 **Miss Hannah Boston**, pauper lunatic from Jackson County, unmarried, age about 50, cause of insanity unknown, duration uncertain, admitted Oct 25ᵗʰ 1849, died of chronic diarrhea complicated with general dropsy 25ᵗʰ May 1850.

240 **Mrs. Sarah Hendrix**, pauper lunatic and epileptic of Lumpkin County, widow, age 38, blind and in bad health, has had epilepsy for 15 years, duration of insanity 6, Oct 27 1849 received, died of atrophy August 20ᵗʰ 1853.

241 **Thos. J. Madrey**, pauper lunatic from Floyd County, age about 35 years, married, farmer, cause of insanity unknown, duration uncertain, admitted Nov 3ʳᵈ 1849.

242 **Col. Gibson Clark**, brother of Gov'r Clark, pauper lunatic from Butts County, age about 70 years, single, lawyer, cause of insanity unknown, duration many years, health very bad, admitted Nov 22 1849, died of chronic diarrhea 1ˢᵗ Feb 1850.

243 **Wm. A. Wright**, a pauper lunatic from Murray County, age about 18, single, farmer, duration of insanity between the recent four years, general health not good, admitted Decr 26ᵗʰ 1849, died Jan 21ˢᵗ 1851.

244 **Darling P. Lee**, pay patient, lunatic from Stewart County, age about 24 years, married (but deserted by wife some three years since) duration of insanity about four years, general health not good, admitted Decr 30ᵗʰ 1849.

245 **Edwin Jones**, pay patient, lunatic from Chattooga County, age 38, married, duration of insanity about one year, general health quite bad, suffering for years with chronic bronchitis, admitted Jany 23ʳᵈ 1850.

246 **John W. Bird**, pay patient, lunatic from Hancock County, age [blank] years, single, duration of insanity [blank] years, general health not very good, admitted Jany 28ᵗʰ 1850, died Oct 25ᵗʰ 1857, address George G. Bird, son of J. W. Bird, Augusta, Georgia.

247 **Jefferson Williams**, pauper patient, lunatic from Forsyth County, age about 35, single, duration of insanity 7 years, health tolerably good, admitted Febry 3ʳᵈ 1850, died 1ˢᵗ Dec 1882.

248 **Thos. D. Robinson**, pay patient from Benton County, Alabama, lunatic, age about 30 years, single, duration of insanity uncertain, once an inmate of the asylum at Columbia, S.C., for 18 months, admitted Feb 22ⁿᵈ 1850, died May 11 1851.

249 **John Brame**, pay patient from Marengo County, Alabama, lunatic, age 20 years, single, duration of insanity about a year, admitted Mar 10ᵗʰ 1850, died Jan 20 1859.

250 **Mrs. Nancy Guest**, pauper lunatic from Cass County, age 33, married, cause of insanity puerperal condition, duration of last attack 4 years, admitted 24ᵗʰ March 1850, died of marasmus July 11ᵗʰ 1851.

251 **Mr. Wm. J. D. Smiley**, ~~pay patient from Crawford County, lunatic, age 33 yrs, single, farmer, cause ill health and disappointed affection, duration of insanity 6 yrs, escaped from this institution Oct 2nd 1847, recommitted and admitted second time Mar 27th 1850, condition much worse than when he escaped.~~

251 **Phineas Terry**, pauper lunatic from Cobb County, age 64, social condition cause and duration of disease unknown, admitted March 29th 1850, died Septr 21 1855.

252 **Wm. Crow**, pauper from Cass County, age 22, single, laborer, cause of disease unknown, duration 5 years, admitted 8th April 1850, died in a paroxysm of convulsions May 7 1852.

253 **John Atcheson**, pauper lunatic from Warren County, age 35, farmer, single, cause of insanity unknown, perhaps ill health, duration several years, admitted 25th Jan 1850, removed by his friends in very much improved condition July 12th 1851. Cured.

254 **Eldridge Cash**, pauper lunatic from DeKalb County, age 36, single, farmer, cause hereditation, duration 15 months, admitted 30th May 1850, removed by his friends Decr. 14th 1850.

255 **Bird Burke**, pauper lunatic from Chatham County, age 40, married, farmer, cause unknown, duration of insanity 15 or 20 years, admitted 2nd June 1850.

256 **Mrs. Margaret Shea**, pauper lunatic from Chatham County, age 30, cause religious excitement, duration 4 months, admitted 2nd day of June 1850, discharged cured 21st Aug 1850.

257 **Feinister Gailey**, pauper lunatic from Hall County, age 24, cause blow upon his head, duration 1 year, single, farmer, admitted 10th June 1850.

258 **Wm. M. Garrow**, lunatic from Mobile, Alabama, pay patient, age 45, cause ill health and peculiarly nervous temperament, duration of last attack 4 or 5 years, married, lawyer, admitted 11th June 1850, removed by his friends 24th June 1850.

259 **Wm. Fergurson, alias Troup**, a congenital pauper, idiot from Randolph County, age 23, admitted 20th December 1849, died of chronic diarrhea May 23rd 1851. This patient was received in 1849 and his name should have been entered with those who came in during that year.

260 **Mrs. Priscilla Kellabrew**, pauper lunatic from Monroe County, age 35, married, mother of six children, farmer, wife cause extreme poverty, duration 8 years, admitted 17th June 1850, died 1 Jan 1892, notified. (Here)

261 **Mary Ann Norris**, pauper idiot and epileptic from Monroe County, age 28, single, cause of epilepsy unknown, duration 15 years, admitted June 17th 1850, died in convulsions March 26th 1851.

262 **Miss Mary Clanton**, lunatic from Macon County, Alabama, pay patient, age 19, cause ill health and loss of mother, duration between 3 and 4 years, admitted 19th June 1852, died 1 Aug 1874, affection liver, notified.

263 **Dulcebella Rogers**, pauper lunatic from Chattooga County, age 29, married, cause loss of property, duration 9 months, admitted 24th June 1850, died Novr 16th 1854.

264 **Mary P. Turner**, lunatic from Hancock County, pay patient, single, age 53 or 4, cause unknown, duration 40 years, admitted to the asylum 24th June 1850. Died.

265 **George W. Farmer**, pauper lunatic form Oglethorpe County, age 45, married, farmer, cause religious excitement, duration 14 months, admitted 28th day June 1850.

266 **Martha Porter**, pauper lunatic from Putnam County, age 35, widow, mother of four or five children, cause of insanity, want, and fear of starvation, duration 2 months, admitted 2nd July 1850, discharged cured Feb 26 1851.

267 **Caroline O. Bryan**, pauper lunatic from Decatur County, age about 40, married, cause and duration of disease unknown, admitted 12th July 1850, removed by her friends Sept 27th 1851.

268 **Mrs. Parthenia E. Mines**, pay patient, lunatic and epileptic from Conecuh County, Alabama, age 24, married, cause ill health with abuse from her husband, duration two years, admitted 13th July 1850, discharged Apl 9th 1856.

269 **Mrs. Jerusha Evans**, pay patient, lunatic from Jones County, age 35, married, cause ill health, together with domestic unhappiness, duration 4 years, admitted 20th July 1850. Died.

270 **Robert T. Allen**, pauper lunatic from Hall County, age 26, single, teacher, cause intense application, duration 3 years, admitted on the 24th day of July 1850, died Augt. 27th 1854.

271 **Cassa Drummond**, pauper lunatic from Walker County, age about 45, single, mother of one or more children, cause, a life of prostitution and want, duration 5 or 6 years, admitted 27th July 1850, died of ascitis May 12th 1851.

272 **Revd. Luke Robinson**, lunatic pay patient from Newton County, age 70, married, cause of insanity ill health and old age, duration 18 months, admitted 5th August 1850, died Feb 13th 1851.

273 **Miss Sophia Barnwell**, pauper lunatic from Savannah, age 25, single, cause not known, duration two years, admitted 21st August 1850, should she die or become seriously sick, notify Mr. Edward W. Barnwell, Guyton, Ga., died 16 Sept 1902, senility. (Here)

274 **Miss Sarah Ann McHugh**, pauper lunatic from Gwinnett County, age 25, single, cause disappointed affection, duration 1 year, admitted 7th Sept 1850, removed improved 7th March 1874. (Here)

275 **Mrs. Amelia E. Pevy**, pauper lunatic from Bibb County, age 25, married, cause abuse from her husband, duration 18 months, admitted 9th Sept 1850, discharged much improved Oct 1st 1851, died Mar 2/55.

276 **Timothy Snelson**, lunatic pay patient from Wilkes County, age 21, single, a clerk, cause hereditation, duration recently, admitted Sept 14th 1850, condition as a pay patient ceased on or about Jany 1st 1851, escaped Feb 8th 1851 [illegible writing]

277 **Matthew Caldwell**, pauper epileptic from Cass County, age 12, single, cause unknown, duration 6 months, admitted Sept 19th 1850, died Apl 27th 1855.

278 **Thomas McGurl**, pauper lunatic from Baldwin County, age about 50, single, ditcher and well digger, cause concussion of the brain, duration 6 or 7 months, admitted Sept 24 1850, died.

279 **Hiram G. Silman**, pauper lunatic from Franklin County, age 33, single, occupation not known, cause of insanity and duration not known, admitted Sept 25th 1850. Died.

280 **Mr. Jonathan Brazil**, pauper idiot from Meriwether County, age 25, single, cause congenital, admitted Sept 27 1850, died of [blank] February 3rd 1853.

281 **Wiley Webb**, pauper lunatic from Meriwether County, age 37, married, cause study and domestic trouble, duration two years or more, admitted Sept 27th 1850, died of typhoid fever July 8th 1851.

282 **Clarissa Hendry**, pauper lunatic from Lowndes County, age 30, married, cause of insanity violent temper, duration about 3 years, admitted Oct 8th 1850, died July 19th 1856.

283 **Katy Kennedy**, pauper lunatic from Union County, age 52, single, cause unknown, duration some 20 or 25 years, admitted Oct 14th 1850, died of phthisis March 28th 1851.

284 **Joseph Johnson**, pauper idiot from Troup County, age 7 years, single, cause congenital, admitted Oct 23rd 1850, died Novr 14 1853.

285 **Margaret Moody**, pauper, lunatic from Meriwether County, age 31, single, cause disappointed affection, duration 6 months, admitted Oct 23 1850, escaped from the institution Dec 10th.

286 **Mrs. Mary M. Wiggens**, lunatic pay patient from Baldwin County, age [blank], married, cause not known, duration [blank], admitted Nov 26 1850, died of remittent fever, complicated with inf[lamation] of bowels and menorrhagia, Sept 16th 1851.

287 **Benjamin T. Chastain**, pauper lunatic from Forsyth County, age 45 or 50, single, duration from early life, admitted Dec 8[th] 1850, died Augt 31[st] 1854.

288 **Mr. Michael Riggle**, pauper lunatic from Cass County, age 55, single, cause unknown, occupation unknown, duration altogether uncertain, admitted Dec 21 1850, died June 20 1854.

289 **Moses Brockman**, pauper lunatic from Clarke County, age 65, widower, cause unknown, occupation waggoner, duration about 8 months, admitted Dec 22[nd] 1850, died July 3[rd] 1852.

290 **Mr. Matheson Henn**, pay patient lunatic from Pike County, Alabama, age about 35, single, cause not known, occupation farmer, duration about 5 years, admitted Dec 25[th] 1850, address Valentine Henn, Indian Creek, Pike County, Alabama, eloped Jan 27[th] 1852, perhaps slightly improved.

291 **Mrs. Milly Parker**, pauper epileptic from Lumpkin County, age 24, married, cause of disease unknown, duration about 5 years, admitted Dec 25[th] 1850.

292 **Mrs. Katharine Reeves**, pauper lunatic from Lumpkin County, age 40, married, cause of lunacy unknown, duration 4 years, admitted Dec 25[th] 1850, died 28 Aug 1855, cholera morbus and old age.

293 **Mr. John Boockout**, pauper lunatic from Cherokee County, age 40, widower, cause of condition not known, duration 7 years, admitted Jan 3[rd] 1851, died of paralysis Jan 19[th] 185[cut off].

294 **Cassandra Curry**, pay patient from Decatur County, age 35, single, cause not known, duration between 16 and 17 years, admitted Jan 16[th] 1851, died of inflammation of the lower bowel, march 18[th] 1854.

295 **Mr. Hezekiah Wassle**, pauper lunatic from Bibb County, age about 28, married, cause intemperance, duration 3 or 4 weeks, admitted Jan 17[th] 1851, discharged cured Feb 17[th] 1851, relapsed and returned to the asylum March 4[th] 1851, again discharged Sept 12[th] 1851.

296 **Frederick G. Clark**, pay patient lunatic from Camden County, age 29, single, cause not known, duration 9 years, admitted Jan 18[th] 1851, died Septr 20 1854.

297 **John Goodson**, pauper partial idiot from Habersham County, age 7 years, condition congenital, admitted Jan 18[th] 1851, died of dysentery with [blank].

298 **Mr. Charles S. Sibley**, pay patient, lunatic from Quincy, Florida, age 40 years, married, cause unknown, occupation lawyer, duration 2 years, admitted Jan 19[th] 1851, removed by his friends June 26[th] 1851, to New Jersey, where his friends resided, placed in asylum at Trenton and died there.

299 **Hunley (alias) Nameless**, pauper lunatic from Muscogee County, age about 35 or 40, cause and duration unknown, admitted Jan 22$^{nd}$ 1851.

300 **Mr. Wily J. Chandler**, pay patient, lunatic from Franklin County, age 20, single, cause of lunacy unknown, duration 4 years, admitted Jan 30$^{th}$ 1851, died Decr 27$^{th}$ 1854.

301 **Mr. James Arnold**, pauper, partial idiot from Stewart County, age about 22, single, condition congenital, admitted Feb 9$^{th}$ 1851, died 1$^{st}$ Aug 1879.

302 **Mr. Bartholomew Arnold**, pauper, partial idiot from Stewart County, age about 20, single, condition congenital, admitted Feb 9$^{th}$ 1851, died of general debility March 18$^{th}$ 1853.

303 **Mrs. Elizabeth A. Powell**, pay patient lunatic from Monroe County, age about 35, married, cause unknown, duration 6 months, admitted Feb 19$^{th}$ 1851, removed by her friends Aug 2$^{nd}$ 1851, died.

304 **Miss Elizabeth Hines**, pay patient, lunatic and epileptic from Decatur County, age about 30, condition of mind congenital, duration of epilepsy 2 years, admitted Feb 20$^{th}$ 1851, died [?]nemia Sept 19$^{th}$ 1851.

305 **Mr. R. B. Hyde**, pay patient, lunatic from Mobile, Alabama, age 35 or 40, cause unknown, duration of insanity recent, admitted Feb 23$^{rd}$ 1851, died of apoplexy July 19$^{th}$ 1851.

306 **Mr. John Broffy**, pauper lunatic from Richmond County, age about 38, single, cause ill health, duration about 1 year, admitted March 11$^{th}$ 1851, died March 24$^{th}$ 1856.

307 **Mrs. Susannah Roney**, of Gordon County, pay patient, married, age 37, lunatic, duration about 1 year, cause uterine disease, admitted Mar 14$^{th}$ 185[cut off].

308 **Mrs. Nancy Jane Douglass**, pauper lunatic from Telfair County, age 27 or 28, married, cause unknown, duration 5 or 6 months, admitted March 18$^{th}$ 1851, died by suicide Aug 13 1851.

309 **Mr. John Ellis**, pauper epileptic from Telfair County, age 28, single, cause of epilepsy unknown, duration 8 or 10 years, admitted March 18$^{th}$ 1851, died in convulsions July 2$^{nd}$ 1852.

310 **John T. Collier**, pauper epileptic from Dooly County, age 11, single, condition congenital, admitted March 22$^{nd}$ 1851, died of a wound on the head, Dec 2$^{nd}$ 1851.

311 **Mr. William Jenkins**, pauper epileptic and idiot from Richmond County, age [blank], admitted March 26$^{th}$ 1851, died Aprl 8$^{th}$ 1854.

312 **Mr. Elijah C. Arthur**, pauper lunatic from Walker County, age about 45, married, cause unknown, duration many years, admitted March 27$^{th}$ 1851, died Sept 20$^{th}$ 1860.

313   **Mr. Robert H. Hale**, pauper lunatic from Walton County, age about 25, single, cause of lunacy ill health, occupation clerk, duration 2 years, admitted March 19[th] 1851, removed by his friends Febry 12 1852, privilege of being returned within one month.

314   **Mrs. Temperance Johnson**, pauper lunatic and epileptic from Gwinnett County, age about 80 years, married, cause unknown, duration of epilepsy 46 years, admitted April 1[st] 1851, died Augt 6[th] 1854.

315   **Miss Mary Stroud**, pauper lunatic from Jasper County, age 85 or 90 years, single, cause of lunacy unknown, duration unknown, admitted April 4[th] 1851, died Jan 20 1852.

316   **Mr. Thomas Johnson**, pauper lunatic from Columbia County, age 25, single, cause disappointed affection, duration two or three weeks, admitted April 5[th] 1851, discharged cured Oct 1[st] 1851.

317   **Mr. Henry K. Demere**, pay patient, lunatic from Bryan County, age 28, single, cause not known, duration 8 years, admitted April 14[th] 1851, eloped April 19[th] 1851 was returned to the institution May 6[th] 1851, eloped Decr 6/57, returned Decr 10/57, eloped Nov 18/74, returned Nov 21/74, eloped 26[th] June 1877, returned 21[st] Sept 1877, address Mr. Raymond Demere, Exchange Building, Savannah, Ga.

318   **Mr. Benj. P. Gray**, pauper lunatic of Henry County, age about 35, single, cause not known, duration uncertain but supposed short time, admitted Apr 17[th] 1851, discharged cured Oct 1[st] 1851.

319   **Mrs. Margarette A. Allen**, pay patient lunatic from Muscogee County, age 18, married, cause of lunacy not known, duration two years, admitted May 1[st] 1851.

320   **Mr. John Caldwell**, pauper lunatic from Muscogee County, age 60, married, cause domestic difficulties, duration about 4 years, admitted May 9[th] 1851, discharged cured Oct 1[st] 1851.

321   **Mr. John D. Hwell** [*sic*], pauper lunatic from Muscogee County, age [blank], married, admitted May 23[rd] 1851.

322   **Mr. Barney Riley**, pauper lunatic from Chatham County, age 32, married, cause of insanity supposed to be jealousy, duration one year, admitted May 27[th] 1851, died Sept. 23[rd] 1854.

323   **Mr. Robert K. Bishop**, pauper lunatic from Harris County, age 41, married, cause of insanity intemperance, duration 25 days, admitted May 27[th] 1851, died of phthisis pulmonalis Sept. 9[th] 1851.

324   **Mr. John Danner**, pauper lunatic and epileptic from Wilkes County, age about 50, married, cause of condition unknown, occupation Baptist preacher, duration of epilepsy 5 years, admitted June 3[rd] 1851.

325   **Mr. Thos. Barnes**, pauper lunatic from Muscogee County, age about 40, other items of history unknown, admitted June 9[th] 1851.

End of year.

326    **Mr. Joab B. Brooks**, pay patient, lunatic from Muscogee County, age 32, single, cause of insanity pecuniary losses and intemperance, duration 4 months, admitted Aug 11[th] 1851, removed by his friends in a much improved condition Nov 4[th] 1851.

327    **Mrs. Elizabeth Dodson**, pauper lunatic from Murray County, age [blank], cause of insanity and duration unknown, admitted Aug 31[st] 1851, died of chronic mania Jan 30[th] 1852.

328    **Mr. F. M. Belcher**, pay patient lunatic from Newton County, age 25, single, cause ill health and hard study, duration about 3 years, admitted Sept 27[th] 1851, died May 12[th] 1858.

329    **Mr. Wm. Boyd**, pauper lunatic from Lumpkin County, age about 60, married, cause ill health and intemperance, duration uncertain, admitted Oct 19[th] 1851, escaped from the institution January 29[th], brought back 30[th], 1853.

330    **Mrs. Jane Gassoway**, pauper lunatic from Cobb County, age 35 or 40, married, cause of insanity ill health, duration about three years, admitted Oct 23[rd] 1851, died Octr 27[th] 1854.

331    **Mrs. Ellen G. Dickson**, pauper lunatic from Baker County, age [blank], married, cause of derangement unknown, duration over a year, admitted Nov 9[th] 1851, died of phthisis pulmonalis April 21[st] 1853.

331    **Miss Mariam Denny**, pauper lunatic from Cass County, age 35, single, cause of insanity unknown, duration 16 years, admitted Nov 12[th] 1851, died 19t July 1909, senility, buried here.

334    **Mrs. Westly Long**, pauper lunatic or idiot from Gilmer County, age about 35, single, other items of information unknown, admitted Nov 24[th] 1851, died of ulceration of the bowels July 7[th] 1853.

335    **Mr. George W. Pritchett**, pay patient from Jasper County, age 21, lunatic, single, cause of insanity unknown, duration about three weeks, admitted Nov 24[th] 1851.

336    **Mr. Wiley Tiner**, pauper lunatic from Lumpkin County, age 50, married, cause unknown, perhaps intemperance, duration a few months, admitted Dec 8[th] 1851, died of collignative diarrhea June 1[st] 1852.

337    **Mrs. Verstille**, pay patient, from Savannah, age about 50, lunatic, married, cause of insanity ill health and religious excitement, duration some months, admitted Jany 16[th] 1852, discharged restored Mar 30[th] 1852.

338    **Lemuel Lovett**, pay patient from Monroe County, about 21, congenital idiot, single, admitted Febry 3[rd] 1852.

339 **A. B. Seals**, pay patient of Enon, Alabama, married, age about 26, discharged from this institution supposed cured on the 6[th] Oct 1845, has been employed almost ever since as a teacher in different important schools until about two weeks back, received Mar 10[th] 1852, removed by his friends without improvement June the 8[th] 1852.

340 **Wm. V. Osborne**, pay patient of Milledgeville, age about 34, single, cause of insanity disappointed affection, duration not known, received May 12[th] 1852.

341 **James W. Winchester**, lunatic pay patient from Heard County, age 22, single, cause loss of brother, duration 33 months, admitted June 21[st] 1852, died of ulceration of the bowels, May 11[th] 185[cut off], address Corinth, Heard County, Ga.

342 **Nancy Smedley**, lunatic from Coweta County, pauper, age about 40, widow, cause of insanity ill health, duration unknown, admitted July 25 1852.

343 **James Smedley**, idiot from Coweta County, child of the above Nancy Smedley, age 7, unnaturally small and deformed, in very bad health, condition congenital, July 25[th] 1852.

344 **Sarah Rohr**, pauper lunatic from Savannah, widow age about 40, cause of insanity death of husband, duration about one year, admitted July 27, 1852.

345 **Robert Duncan**, pauper lunatic from Gwinnett County, age 30, single, cause of insanity unknown, duration seven years, left the asylum in Columbia S. Carolina two years previous, in a condition favorable to his restoration, admitted September 15[th] 1852.

346 **John Copeland**, pauper lunatic and epileptic from Cobb County, age 24, single, cause of lunacy is said to be the taking of quinine, duration 3 or 4 years, admitted Sep 9[th] 1852.

347 **John Jenkins**, pauper lunatic from Green County, age 27, married, cause hereditary and religious study, duration 2 to 6 months, occupation printer, his health previous to the first symptoms of insanity was remarkably good, admitted November 11[th] 1852.

351 **Henry M. Jernigan**, admitted Febry 23[rd] 1852.

352 **Mrs. Mangum**, admitted Augt 12 1852.

353 **Miss E. Kellum**, admitted August 17, 1852.

354 **Miss Margaret L. Pollard**, admitted August 19 1852.

355 **Margaret Henderson**, admitted August 23 1852.

356 **Daniel Ashford**, admitted June 10 1852.

348  **N. Y. Espy**, pauper idiot from Spalding County, age 16, cause of present condition congenital, was deformed from birth and is now perfectly helpless, admitted January 17[th] 1853, died of diarrhea April 29[th] 1853.

349  **Virginia Florence**, pauper idiot from Lincoln County, single, age 22, condition congenital, never violent or distinctive, not careful in her personal habits, often soils her cloths, admitted March 4[th] 1853, died of colliquative diarrhea October 21[st] 1853.

350  **John W. Johnson**, pauper lunatic from Forsyth County, age about 25, single, occupation student of law, cause of present condition hard study, duration 1 year, no hereditary predisposition traceable, is not violent, temperate in his habits, nine months ago shot his father and killed him, admitted March 5[th] 1853.


[The following appears within the index between H and M, found at the conclusion of the volume.]

S. V. Kelly left the institution on the 28 June, returned 10 July. S. V. Kelly left institution 31[st] July, returned 31 August, returned on the 3[rd] at ½ past 3 and left for Milledgeville at 5 o'clock.

Mr. Stembridge left the institution 13[th] Aug and returned Aug 17.

T. J. Micklejohn left August 24 and returned 25[th].

Mr. Watson employed Aug 28[th].

Raiford left for Houston, Oct 6[th], returned to asylum Oct 10[th].

Mr. Leonard eumployed Oct 22 1853 as an attendant in 2[nd] galley.

Raiford about Saturday from [?] o'clock at home, the 27 Oct to [?] with his wife.

23 Oct Raiford absent ½ day with his boy Barney.

9 Nov absent from 10 AM during the day.

# Volume 2: 1853–1861

356  **Miss Martha McRae**, lunatic, pay patient from Montgomery County, age 21, single, causes excessive use of tobacco and hereditary predisposition, duration about 9 months, admitted March 26th 1853, discharged cured October 1st 1853.

357  **Joseph E. H. Newton**, lunatic, pay patient from Clarke County, age 18, single, cause supposed to be the structure of the urethra, duration 1 year but more particularly noticeable 8 months ago, admitted April 6th 1853, discharged much improved October 1st 1853.

358  **William P. Winters**, pauper lunatic from Jackson County, age 32, married, occupation farmer, cause of present condition hereditary, duration four years, but indications more decidedly obvious for the past six months, since which his general health has grown rapidly worse, has not been violent, is filthy in his habits, admitted April 16th 1851, died of chronic diarrhea March 28th 1854.

359  **Daniel McCook**, pauper lunatic and epileptic from Hancock County, age [blank], married, farmer, cause of present condition epileptic convulsions, which have existed ever since he was five years, generally quiet and orderly, paroxysms occur twice a month at the full and change of the moon as he states, admitted April 18th 1853, died December 2nd 1855.

360  **William Wilson**, pauper lunatic, transferred from the penitentiary, having been convicted of simple larceny in the Superior Court of Cobb County, under certificate of the penitentiary physician, age about 35, remained in the penitentiary three weeks, admitted Apr 21st 1853, removed from the asylum back to the penitentiary April 29, 1853.

361  **John Crawford**, pauper lunatic and epileptic from Newton County, age 20 years, single, cause of present condition unknown, duration 12 years, paroxysms occur at irregular intervals, and is violent at times, admitted April 25th 1853, died of marasmus December 5th 1853.

362  **William Hyde**, pauper lunatic from DeKalb County, age about 23 years, single, laborer, cause of derangement perjury, duration 1 year 3 months but became decidedly insane 6 months ago, is not violent nor filthy in his habits, admitted May 4 1853, address Alexr. McDonald, East Point, Fulton County, died December 12, 1857.

363  **Martin Baker**, pauper lunatic from Marion County, age about 40 years, widower, farmer, cause of insanity religious study, duration about 7 years, is not filthy in his habits, admitted May 5th 1853, died of marasmus Nov 11th 1853.

364  **Malachi J. Frost**, pauper lunatic and epileptic from Walker County, age 20, single, occupation laborer, cause of present condition epileptic convulsions, duration from early youth, admitted May 5th 1853, died August 6 1854.

365 **Samuel L. Ward**, pauper from Whitfield County, age about 45, married, farmer, cause of derangement domestic trouble and intemperance, duration 15 years, is noisy and mischievous, but not violent, admitted May 6th 1853, discharged cured Oct 1st 1853.

366 **Samuel Boyd**, congenital idiot, part paying patient from Spalding County, age 30, single, although ordinarily passive and quiet, yet is sometimes violent towards children and females, admitted May 24th 1853, died June 4th 1854.

367 **Isabella H. Richards**, lunatic and epileptic, pay patient from Bibb County, age 14, cause of epilepsy a blow on the head from a fall, which blow she received when two years old, followed by convulsions which lasted three days, from that time she did not experience another attack of convulsions until the expiration of one year when they reoccurred and have continued every since at irregular intervals, admitted June 16th 1853, died April 1st 1855.

368 **Louiza Harrington**, pauper lunatic from Harris County, age about 30, cause of lunacy unknown, duration 6 or 7 years, admitted June 20th 1853, died of ulceration of the bowels, May 5th 1854.

369 **Henderson Poteete**, pauper lunatic from Union County, age 45, married, farmer, cause of derangement intemperance and trouble, duration about 14 months, but more particularly noticeable 6 months ago, admitted July 3rd 1853, died Sept 23 1854.

370 **Mr. J. C. Huff**, pauper lunatic from Warren County but when committed he resided in Jefferson County, age 27, single, farmer, cause over [heat?] connected with trouble, duration 2 years 7 months, admitted July 10th 1853, address Mrs. J. W. Lee, 49 Edwards St, Atlanta, address 9-30-1901 Mrs. M. E. Pentecost, Gadsden, Ala., died 29 Dec 1901, apoplexy.

371 **Sarah Scarborough**, pauper lunatic from Pulaski County, age about 50, married, cause of derangement ill health, duration about 3 years, is violent at times making attempts to commit murder, admitted July 12th 1853.

372 **Mrs. Mary A. Lunsay**, lunatic pay patient from Bibb County, age 24, married, has 3 children, cause of present condition uterine disease connected with domestic trouble, duration 1 year, though no decided manifestations were apparent until 7 months ago, admitted July 17th 1853, removed by her husband much improved October 8th 1853, admitted again June 6 1857.

373 **William Brockett**, pauper lunatic from Baker County, age 45, married, farmer and trader, cause of derangement syphilis connected with loss of property, duration about 3 months, admitted July 21st 1853, discharged cured Nov 25 1854.

374 **John Lard**, pauper lunatic from Newton County, age 32, single, occupation overseer on plantation, cause of derangement a blow on the head, duration 6 years, but more decided manifestations of derangement

have been apparent about 1 year, admitted July 25[th] 1853, died 6[th] May 173, marasmus.

375  **Mary A. Hubbard**, lunatic pay patient from Richmond County, age 43, married, has five children, cause of derangement loss of son, duration about 7 years, was removed from the Columbia Asylum S. Carolina 8 months ago having remained in that institution 2 years without having undergone any material change, admitted Aug 13[th] 1853, discharged cured Oct 1[st] 1856, having relapsed was again received Jan 26 1858.

376  **Thomas Busby**, pauper idiot from Houston County, age 26, a hereditary disposition traceable, admitted August 11[th] 1853, died of marasmus April 30[th] 1854.

377  **Benjamin Busby**, pauper idiot from Houston County, age 21, a hereditary predisposition traceable, admitted August 11[th] 1853, died suddenly the 20[th] October 1853.

378  **Joseph Busby**, pauper idiot from Houston County, age 12, a hereditary predisposition traceable, admitted August 11[th] 1853, died 26 Oct 1897, shock from operation.

379  **Wesley Johnson**, pauper lunatic from Clinch County, age 44, married, farmer, cause of present condition jealousy of wife, duration 14 months, admitted August 13[th] 1853, discharged cured Oct 1[st] 1853.

380  **John Bowman**, pauper epileptic idiot from Murray County, age 20, cause of epilepsy a blow on the head, duration 4 years, admitted September 13[th] 1853, died Jan 29 1854.

381  **John R. Daniel**, pauper lunatic from Emanuel County, age 62, married but has been separated from his wife fifteen or twenty years, occupation saddler, cause unknown, duration 15 years, admitted September 24[th] 1853, died of paralysis Oct 13 1856.

382  **Frederick K. Taylor**, lunatic pay patient from Jefferson County, age 22, single, school teacher, cause of present condition irritation from stone in the bladder connected with religious excitement, duration 6 or 8 months, admitted September 30[th] 1853, discharged cured August 31 1854.

383  **William Ethridge**, pauper lunatic from Randolph County, age 21, single, occupation working on a farm, cause of present condition religious excitement, duration about 2 months, admitted October 12[th] 1853, discharged cured February 8[th] 1854.

384  **Elias Lee**, lunatic pay patient from Early County, age 35, married, farmer, cause of present condition domestic trouble and the excessive use of tobacco, duration 5 months, admitted Oct 30[th] 1853, discharged cured Feb 10[th] 1854, readmitted August 4[th] 1854, readmitted under new commitment Sept 1 instead of August 1, discharged April 14 1855, received again November 27, 1857.

385 **Timothy Murphy** (Irishman), pauper lunatic from Monroe County, age 29, single, occupation ditcher and stone mason, cause unknown, duration 3 months, admitted Sep 2nd 1853, died 7 Mar 1892, influenza. Notified.

386 **Mrs. Winfred J. Stapp**, lunatic pay patient from Pickens County, Alabama, age 26, widow, with one child about 9 months old, cause of present condition loss of relations, duration 1 year 1 month, but decided manifestations of derangement not observed until a month ago when she exhibited some suicidal tendency, has not attempted any serious injury to other persons, she is in feeble general health, admitted Nov 16th 1853, discharged cured May 7 1855, address C. M. Fort, Pickensville, Ala.

387 **Mrs. Polly A. Floyd**, pauper lunatic and epileptic from Hall County, age 36, widow, cause of present condition epileptic convulsions, duration unknown, admitted Nov 18th 1853.

388 **Miss Lucinda McPherson**, epileptic and lunatic from Gwinnett County, partial pay patient, age 35, unmarried, duration of disease 25 years, admitted Decr 20 1853, died Nov 23 1858.

389 **Mrs. Nancy Blount**, pauper lunatic from Pike County, age about 50, married, cause hereditary tendency and the critical period of life, duration about three months, third attack, admitted Jany 10th 1854, address G. B. M. Blount, Flat Shoals, Meriwether County, removed by her husband much improved April 29th 1854.

390 **Mrs. King H. Mullens**, lunatic pay patient from Stewart County, age 33, married with 5 children, farmer, causes exciting jealousy, predisposing hereditary, duration 11 months, but more particular manifestations of derangement have been exhibited one month and a half, admitted December 14th 1853, died Oct 21 1854.

391 **Mr. William Moss**, pauper lunatic from Henry County, age 51, cause hereditary tendency, duration of present attack unknown, this is the third attack, the 1st lasted 12 or 14 months and in the second attack when derangement had existed for two months was brought to this institution and remained for 3 months when he recovered and was discharged from the asylum, Aug 1st 1859, admitted Jan 12th 1854, address Melissa Moss, Flat Rock, Henry County, discharged recovered June 15th 1854.

392 **Miss Emily Hardwike**, lunatic part pay patient from Newton County, age 27 or 8, single, supposed cause ill health, duration three years, sometimes exhibits a disposition to acts of violence towards others, never towards herself, is disposed to set fire to her clothes and other things and sometimes destroys clothing and bedding by tearing up, admitted February 3rd 1854.

393 **Mr. Richard Felton**, lunatic pay patient from Cobb County, age 64, married the second time, farmer and carpenter, cause of present condition a blow on the head producing fracture of the bone with depression, duration between 6 and 7 months, but began to exhibit decided symptoms

of derangement 3 months ago by being refractory and unmanageable and seeking to do acts of violence to his best friends, admitted February 4[th] 1854, died Jan 21[st] 1855.

394    **Mr. William M. Potter**, pauper lunatic from Early County, age 25, single, teacher, preacher, cause of derangement hard study, duration between two and three years, admitted Feb 11[th] 1854, discharged cured Oct 23 1854.

395    **Mr. William Reed**, pauper lunatic from Murray County, age 26, single, laborer, cause of present condition unknown, duration 18 months, is peaceably disposed, though frequently noisy, general health better than it has been for the past two years, admitted February 17[th] 1854, discharged cured Octr 23[rd] 1854. Readmitted.

396    **Mr. Philip Kean** (Irishman), from Chatham County, age [blank], married, cause of present condition [blank], duration [blank], admitted Febry 22[nd] 1854, address his wife Eliza M. Kean or his brother Edward Kean, Savannah, Ga. Son in law Mr. A. L. Sellman, Macon, Ga.

397    **William Drake**, pauper lunatic and epileptic from Whitfield County, age 17, cause of present condition epileptic convulsions which was produced from a blow on the head producing fracture of the skull, duration for several years, he is not violent nor filthy in his habits, admitted Feb 28[th] 1854, died Oct 29 1854.

398    **Mr. John Hatch**, lunatic pay patient from Cass County, age 52, married to second wife, farmer, cause of present condition domestic trouble, duration 6 months, but decided manifestations of derangement apparent only 2 months, admitted March 2[nd] 1854, died of maniacal exhaustion May 1[st] 1854, address Mr. Jno D. Hatch, Cassville.

399    **Mr. Isaac Seabolt**, pauper lunatic from Lumpkin County, age 36, married, farmer, cause of present condition jealousy, duration 2 years, admitted March 10[th] 1854, died 22 June 1904, apoplexy, address Mrs. Barbara A. Seabolt, Loudsville, White County, Ga., address Berry Turner, Pleasant Retreat, Lumpkin County, address 11-1898 Mr. Geo. W. Seabolt, Pleasant Retreat, Ga.

400    **Mr. Brison Kennedy**, pauper lunatic from Dade County, age 19, single, laborer, cause of present condition an attack of fever affecting his head, duration 2 years 6 months, destroys clothing and bedding by tearing up, noisy and disposed to do acts of violence towards others, admitted Mar 23[rd] 1854, discharged May 10 1855.

401    **Mr. Henry Smith**, lunatic pay patient from Tattnall County, age 73, married, farmer, cause of derangement religious study, duration 1 year 3 months, but decided manifestations of derangement apparent only 6 months, has on several occasions threatened and made attempts to do violence to his family, never to himself, is decent in his person but noisy and troublesome, especially at night, admitted April 6[th] 1854, died of dysentery and probably ulcerations of the bowels existed June 18[th] 1854.

402  **Mr. Bennet Lemasters**, pauper lunatic and epileptic from Troup County, age 30, married, farmer, cause of present condition epileptic convulsions, supposed cause of epilepsy hard work, duration of convulsions 7 years, but mind seriously affected for 1 year, recently made attacks upon his father and other relatives, struck his father and injured him, some convulsions occur irregularly both in the night and day, admitted April 8th 1854, died August 3rd 1855.

403  **Mr. F. S. Cunningham**, pauper lunatic from Cobb County, age 55, married, farmer, cause unknown, duration about 2 months, he has suicidal tendencies having four days ago struck himself in the head with a hoe, his general health appears to be impaired, admitted April 21st 1854, died after three days sickness June 18th 1854.

404  **Mrs. Julia A. Ray**, lunatic pay patient from Morgan County, age 21, married, has one child, cause puerperal, duration 3 months, admitted April 24th 1854, discharged cured June 20 1854.

405  **Mr. James J. Howell**, pauper lunatic and epileptic from Monroe County, age 35, married, has four children, farmer, cause of derangement epileptic convulsions, duration of epilepsy unknown, duration of derangement 5 months, seeks to offer violence to others, never to himself, is not filthy in his habits, admitted May 3rd 1854, died Feb 23 1855.

406  **Mr. John Bunyan Cook**, lunatic pay patient from Baldwin County, age 22, single, farmer, cause religious study, duration 7 months, but more decided indications became apparent 2 months ago, does not seek for opportunities to destroy his own life, but manifests a reckless indifference for his own safety, admitted May 5th 1854, discharged cured Oct 23rd 1854, readmitted Feb 11th 1851 from Texas, address J. M. Cook, Dangerfield, Titus Co, Texas, causes of relapse indolence and self pollution.

407  **Eugene Gavan**, pauper lunatic from Bibb County, received May 22nd 1854, discharged cured April 2nd 1855, readmitted Jan 30 1858, discharged cured Sept 1858.

408  **Mr. Wright Scoggins**, pauper lunatic from Randolph County, age 35, supposed married, wife and 2 children, farmer, cause of insanity unknown, duration about 18 months, no suicidal tendency, manifests a disposition to do violence to others when attempts to control him are made, not destructive, is neat and cleanly, general health not good, admitted May 28th 1854.

409  **Mrs. Caroline Todd**, pauper lunatic from Gwinnett County, age 28, married, having 4 living children, cause of derangement child bearing connected with violent passion, duration 4 years, admitted May 29th 1854, died Feb 17 1855.

410  **Mr. Thomas Bullard**, pauper lunatic from Cobb County, age 24, married, farmer, cause of present condition religious study, duration of derangement 2 months, has made attempts to do others injury, but never

to himself, is not filthy in his habits, but he is occasionally noisy, admitted June 6th 1854, died Dec 9th 1859.

411   **Mr. William H. Thompson**, pauper lunatic from Houston County, age 26, single, overseer, supposed cause ill health, duration of derangement 2 years, he is mischievous and troublesome, six or seven weeks ago became very uncontrollable, so much that his friends had to confine him in jail, admitted June 23rd 1854, eloped Apl 17/57, retd Apl 26/57, died of [blank] Nov 17 1857.

412   **Wm. Johnson**, pauper idiot from Bibb County, 35 years, single, condition congenital, general health rather feeble, usually quiet and tractable, disposed to aid in carrying wood and water and in minding stock, admitted July 17th 1854, died Sept 29 1856

413   **James Jenkins**, pauper lunatic from Richmond County, married, age about 32, duration of insanity unknown, cause hereditation, two brothers previously here, general health tolerably good, occupation printer, admitted July 20th 1854.

414   **Wm. Philips**, pauper lunatic and epileptic from Emanuel County, married, age about 40, duration and cause unknown, general health very imperfect, occupation farmer, admitted July 20th 1854, died May 31st 1855.

415   **Nancy J. Black**, pauper lunatic and epileptic from Effingham County, single, age about 15 years, duration of disease less than one year, supposed cause [Amenorhoea?] and hereditation, father a partial idiot, occupation ordinary domestic duties of her father's cabin, admitted July 23rd 1854, died Sept 24 1855.

416   **Mary Elard**, pauper lunatic from Forsyth County, age [blank], duration and cause unknown, single, admitted July 22n 1854, died 8 Aug 1904, [organic?] heart disease, 1887 Mr. A. J. Key, cor. North Avenue and Orme Sts, Atlanta, Ga.

417   **Mrs. Olive Littlejohn**, pauper lunatic from Greene County, widow, age about 70, duration of disease about 3 years, supposed cause the death and clandestine dissection of her daughter and subsequent circumstances attending it, admitted July 24th 1854, died Sept 29 1854.

418   **James W. Norman**, partial pay patient from Marion County, married, age 32, duration 4 years, supposed cause ill health, occupation farmer, admitted Aug 2nd 1854, died Nov 24th 1858, address Danl Majors, Glenalta, Marion Co.

419   **Mrs. Jane Allen**, pay patient from Spalding County, widow, age 60, duration became insane some twenty years back, or more, and has never been regarded as altogether sound at any time since, but not in such circumstances as to make it necessary to restrain her until some two years back, cause unknown, general health quite feeble, admitted Aug 2nd 1854. If she dies in the institution we have promised that her body shall be

sent in a metallic burial case to the address of Edward Foster or A. S. Allen, Griffin. Discharged cured but in feeble health May the 5[th] 1853.

420 **Isaiah Attaway**, pay patient from near Tuskegee, Alabama, married, age 52, duration about 17 years, supposed cause, hereditation, occupation farmer, admitted Aug 2[nd] 1854, discharged 14 August 1856. Readmitted Aug 22 1856, second admission, he having been an inmate of the asylum (living then in Twiggs Co, Geo) and discharged then, because of the failure of his friends to supply the means for payment of his board &c., discharged March 9[th] 1857.

421 **Wm. Reynolds**, pauper lunatic and epileptic from Decatur County, age and duration or cause all unknown to the party bringing him to the asylum, married, admitted Aug 10[th] 1854, died Sept 6 1854.

422 **Miss Penelope T. Carswell**, pay patient from Houston County, single, age about 32, duration of disease uncertain, indications of derangement occasionally observed for several years, but of most decided character for two years or more, supposed cause loss of property, disappointed affection, with subsequent imprudence use of medicine and snuff, admitted Aug 19[th] 1854, removed according to advice of Supt. Aug 10 1854.

423 **Miss Sarah E. Bashler**, pauper idiot of Bryan County, age about 15, condition congenital, admitted Aug 23, 1854.

424 **Mrs. Missouri J. P. Bell**, pauper patient from DeKalb County, married, at 20, three children, age 25, epileptic 10 years, duration of lunacy about 1 year, admitted Sept 4 1854, died Sept 23[rd] 1860, address John White, Panthersville, DeKalb Co.

425 **Lucinda Wilson**, pauper patient from Cass County, epileptic and idiotic, duration and causes unknown, supposed to have been epileptic from infancy, admitted Sept the 7[th] 1854, disch. Nov 29 1854.

426 **Mrs. Mary J. Daly**, pay patient from Augusta, married, age 25 or 26, has three children, last child in his fifth year, no pregnancy since that birth of that child, was on a visit to the parents of her husband in Ireland two years back when the earliest indications were observed of this tendency to lunacy, when she first visited Ireland her health was very delicate, remaining there one year, she recovered her health and returned at its expiration "stout and fleshy," after her return she remained in a state of depression and seemed indifferent to her children and household affairs, this state continued with little change up to March 1854 when she became violent, eat very little and had many strange decisions upon the subject of religion, being a Catholic in march last she was taken to the Mount Hope Asylum for the Insane in Maryland where she remained four months, then she was removed unimproved, has continued at home since, has never committed any act of violence upon herself or any one else, but sometimes threatened to kill herself, often asks that others would kill her, has never been subject to personal restraint, her general health apparently pretty good appetite, does not sleep well, primary cause supposed

jealousy, admitted Sept 14[th] 1854, Oct 9[th] 1856 removed by friend, Nov 21[st] 1856 readmitted, removed last time June 29[th] 1861.

427 **W. S. Tarpley**, pauper patient from Wilkinson County, single, age about 36, duration supposed five or six years, cause loss of property and friends, admitted Sept 20 1854.

428 **Elizabeth Miles**, pauper lunatic from Upson County, age 60, husband been dead about eight years, the mother of eight children, duration of lunacy about 8 years, cause unknown, present state feeble and complains much, partially blind, admitted 27 Sept 1854, died 9[th] May 1877, old age. Notified.

429 **Robert Hurt**, pay patient from Jackson County, Alabama, married, age about 30, he has been engaged in farming until within the last two years, during which time he has been attending to no business nor has he been capable, about 6 years ago he removed to Mississippi and settled upon the Yazoo River where he suffered from a severe attack of fever followed by inflammation of spleen and liver, first symptoms of mental imbecility were manifested during treatment of and recovery from this attack, his mind becoming impressed with the idea that his medical attendants were attempting to kill him by administering poison, this with other delusions of a similar kind was prominently manifested and fully developed upon his return to Alabama, which took place more than two years ago, and has continued to increase up to present time, he has never exhibited any violence, only towards his brother-in-law who he believes is trying to swindle him and also deprive him of his wife, he is still resolutely determined upon committing this act, has been confined and was brought here bound under false premises, he is restly [restless] and uneasy, believing that those about wish to kill him, admitted 2[nd] Oct 1854, removed 12[th] May 1875, improved.

430 **Loyd A. Knight**, pauper lunatic from Coweta County, occupation physician, married, age 25, duration of lunacy near [?] years, cause said to be intense application to study, lunacy [?] [?], violent particularly towards those who have him charge, attempts to injure by hurling stones etc., prior to his attack friendly sociable and communicative, now silent, morose and sullen, disposed to isolate himself, temperate, is at present laboring under disorder of digestive functions consequent upon an attack of [ferm?], lunacy hereditary, mother now insane, admitted Oct 11 1854, address J. M. Crouch, Bear Creek, Henry Co.

431 **Frances Bohannon**, pauper lunatic from Ware County, married, age 27 years, mother of four children, causes of lunacy but supposed [?] and ill treatment by her husband rendered her condition worse, duration 4 years, admitted October 14 1854, died June 7[th] 1862.

432 **Willis Lord**, pauper idiot from Fayette County, congenital, age 36, admitted Oct 14 1854, died August 25 1857.

433 **Bethena Lord**, pauper idiot from Fayette County, sister of the above, congenital, age 33, admitted Oct 14 1854, died May 21$^{st}$ 1855.

434 **Elizabeth Gully**, pauper idiot from Clarke County, congenital, age about 28, admitted Oct 19 1854.

435 **Charity Gully**, pauper idiot from Clarke County, congenital, age about 26, admitted Oct 19 1854, died June 22 1855.

436 **Lourancy L. Wood**, pauper lunatic from Gwinnett County, duration 20 years, causes supposed deranged catamenies [catamenia], age 40, general health pretty good, admitted Oct 21 1854.

437 **Mathew Kelly**, pauper epileptic from Twiggs County, causes unknown, duration three years, paroxysms frequent, has been intemperate, age about 50, health at present bad, pale and feeble, mind feeble, has never been under treatment, not violent, no restraint necessary, admitted Nov the 8 1854.

438 **Jos. Dubberly**, pay patient from Tattnall County, lunatic age 60, causes religious excitement, duration six years, sometimes violent, attempted suicide by cutting his throat with a razor, admitted Nov 8, 1854, died Oct 13 1855.

439 **Nicholas Nelson**, pauper patient from Early County, age 69, duration of lunacy fifteen years, causes intemperance, particularly delusions, supposes he is "haunted," has never been confined or subjected to any treatment, general health feeble, constitution enfeebled and rendered cachestic by intemperance, admitted Nov 15 1854, died July 18, 1857.

440 **Matilda Trussel**, pauper patient from Early County, age 26, married, one child, duration 18 months, cause "jealousy," admitted Nov 15 1854.

441 **Alexander King**, pay patient from Sumter County, age 20, duration 5 weeks (to some extend 5 years), causes phrenology and [?] [?] [?], he is restless, tears his clothes and any thing he can get hold of, admitted Nov 12 1854, discharged cured June 19 1855.

442 **Shadrach James**, pauper lunatic from Thomas County, age about 22, single, duration about 5 months, causes supposed to be disappointed and misplaced affection, disease increasing, he has intervals of partial reason, intervals shorter and less frequent, not violent, does not try to injure himself or others, has been confined for two months in jail, disease hereditary, his mother and aunt being at the present time lunatics, temperate and free from bad habits, been subjects to no treatment, admitted Nov 18 1854, discharged cured Oct 1$^{st}$ 1855.

443 **John A. C. Knowles**, pauper from Dooly County, farmer, duration six weeks, lunacy first manifested by talking and wandering from place to place, causes supposed to be religious excitement, disease increasing, at times very violent, disposed to fight, very destructive to clothes, glass etc.,

filthy in his habits, temperate, constitution scrupulous, admitted Nov 25 1854, died July 19 1855.

444 **Mary A. M. Murray**, pay patient from Columbia County, age 36, duration 18 years, causes supposed to result from a severe attack of inflammation of the brain, no particular delusions, not disposed to injure himself or others, sometimes destructive to clothes etc, has been treated by several different medical men without the slightest benefit, admitted Decbr 5[th] 1854, died Mar 2[nd] 1861.

445 **George M. Crews**, pay patient from Harris County, age 13, duration 8 years, causes supposed to be the result of a friend occasioned by an animal show, admitted December 9[th] 1854, address Dr. C. C. Crews, [Grenbill?] off., Stewart Co.

446 **Wesley Sanders**, pauper patient from Warren County, idiot, admitted Dec 12 1854.

447 **Mrs. Maria F. Osborne**, admitted December 14 1854, died June 2[nd] 1855.

448 **Dr. Jesse Kirby**, admitted Dec 14 1854, from Morgan County, died Jan 11 1907, senile gangrene, buried here, address 1886, his son Mr. A. J. Kirby, Silver City, New Mexico, address 1890 Dec 8, Mrs. M. J. Hough, Oxford, Ga., address 11-13-05 Mr. J. M. Keith, Mt. Pleasant, Tex.

449 **John C. Rhodes**, pauper lunatic from DeKalb County, age 23, causes unknown, supposed to be the effect of dropsy, is violent, destructive to clothing, glass, etc, uncleanly in his habits, health bad, constitution chachective [cachetic], laboring at present under derangement of hepative function [hepatic system], duration 4 years, admitted January 5[th] 1855, died Oct 3[rd] 1855.

450 **Cinthia Dorough**, pay patient from Upson County, age 34, duration of insanity about 6 weeks, first symptoms manifested on returning home from a visit and finding her house on fire believing that her children were consumed, has been confined to prevent her from setting fire to houses etc, tendency hereditary, heath bad, 4 children, impaired menstrual function, admitted Jan 5 1853, discharged cured April 2[nd] 55.

451 **Wiley J. Shepard**, pauper epileptic and lunatic from Wilkinson County, age about 21 years, duration 12 years, disposed to be violent to himself as well as others, admitted January 8[th] 1855, if he should die inform Wm. Sheppard McDonald, off. Wilkinson Co., Central R.R., will remove his remains, died August 13[th] 1855.

452 **Michael Higgins**, pauper patient from Bibb County, received January 18 1855, age about 16 years, came within the past 8 months from Ireland, duration of insanity two months, cause unknown, occupation ditcher, general health pretty good, temperate, disposed to offer violence to others, admitted January 18 1855, died May 1855 [date of death 1[?], the second number overwritten with 1, 7, and 8].

453 **Mrs. Mary Crosby**, pay patient from Conecuh County, Alabama, age about 30, married, but separated from her husband, the mother of four children, youngest child fourteen years, first attack of insanity occurred four years ago and continued with rational interval for 12 months or more, then she seemed to fully recover her mind, remained pretty well with occasional aberration of mind until about 4 months ago when she became decidedly insane, cause of first attack supposed to be loss of children together with ill treatment upon the part of her husband, of last attack no appreciable or known cause, violent, destructive to clothes etc, general health good, disease hereditary *her mother*, admitted January 25 1855, discharged cured April 23rd 1856.

454 **Mrs. Maria Flannigan**, patient from Cherokee County, age about 40, married but has never borne children, lunacy occurred about 10 or 15 years ago, the effect of epilepsy to which she is now subject, convulsions occurring every night, suffering from deranged catamenia prolapsus uterus, admitted February the 15 1855, died March 22nd 1855.

455 **Benjamin H. Burton**, pauper lunatic from Franklin County, age 36, married, farmer, first symptoms manifested 8 years ago, decided insanity occurred about 6 yrs ago, disease increasing, no particular delusions, his health is not good, is suffering from partial paralysis of lower extremities, locomotion very difficult, has suffered much from syphilis, is at times very violent and unmanageable, tries to injure those that come about him, destructive to clothing and every thing in his reach, never attempts to injure himself, is very filthy in his habits, has been very intemperate in his use of women and whiskey, disease hereditary, his mother at the present is insane, admitted March the 3rd 1855, address Jane Burton, Carnesville, Franklin Co., died August 30 1855.

456 **DeWit C. Morgan**, pay patient from DeKalb County, age 17, duration seven days, first symptoms discoverable about 14 days ago, his condition is one of extreme excitement, raving, hallowing, cursing, kicking, violent, destructive to everything, causes of disease not known, the death of his father supposed to have had some effect, his health to some extent is impaired, has just undergone depletory treatment, has had slight hemorrhage from lung, predisposed to pulmonary disease by hereditary transmission, father died with phthisis pulm., admitted March the 19th 1855, discharged cured.

457 **Sarah Sosebee**, pauper lunatic from Habersham County, age 35 yrs, married, 4 children, youngest 20 months old, first symptoms were manifested 10 years ago, became decidedly insane 8 years ago, has [?] intervals, causes unknown, believes she "is called to preach," health pretty good, has been subjected to treatment for insanity, not violent, destructive to clothing etc, never tries to injure herself or anyone, admitted March 11 1855, died Augt 7th 1861.

458 **Sally Sosebee**, pauper lunatic from Habersham County, age about 30, single, duration 8 years, causes and history of disease unknown, health

good, not violent but destructive to clothing, will fight but does not try to injure herself, a total obliteration of intellect, admitted March the 11[th] 1855, for Sarah Sosebee, address Elias Sosebee, Bushville, Franklin Co., for Sally, Thomas Sosebee, Nacoochee, Habersham.

459 **Mrs. Margeret Conway**, died 28 July 1894, old age, do not notify Ordinary. Jany 15 1887 (grandmother) Mr. R. H. Conway c/s/ U.S. Marshall, Savannah, Ga. Jany 25 1887, Mr. M. A. Henkel, Winter Park, Fla. 5-3-94, Miss Maria Conway, 55 Jefferson St, Savannah, Ga.

460 **John C. Reed**, pay patient from Hart County, age 25, single, farmer, duration 9 months, earliest manifestations about 12 months ago, causes violent attack pneumonia with the loss by death of his mother and brother, sometimes violent, destructive to his clothing etc, has never been subjected to any treatment, has been confined to prevent his killing or hurting his family, was brought to the institution in chains, admitted March 29[th] 1855, address George Reed, Parkers Store, discharged Octr 6[th] 1855.

461 **Sally Creamer**, pauper lunatic from Walker County, age about 35, duration 6 months, causes unknown but supposed bad health, has three children, youngest 9 months old, she has been subjected to medical treatment, not violent, has tried to destroy herself by jumping into a well, also by cutting off her toes in order to bleed herself to death, admitted April 23[rd] 1853, address J. W. Creamer, Lafayette, Walker Co.

462 **Nancy Davis**, pauper lunatic from Spalding County, age about 35, married, six children, youngest 7 years, duration seven years, cause unknown, supposed to be puerperal, prominent delusion hatred to her husband and relations, general health good, habits filthy, destructive to clothing, sometimes violent and threatens to ill, has been treated for disease, admitted 24 April 1855, died Mar 18/56.

463 **Nancy Carpenter**, pauper lunatic from Upson County, single, age 40 years, first symptoms manifested ten years ago, decidedly insane 8 years ago, causes unknown, disease hereditary, no prominent delusions, is not apparently in a state of dementia, general health had broken arm, has elephantiasis, destructive to clothing, habits filthy, does not try to injure herself, but often attempts to kill others etc., admitted April 24 1855, died June 30 1855.

464 **John Sprayberry**, pauper patient from Chattooga County, age 26, single, farmer, duration 6 years, causes unknown, prominent traits consist in mistaken views upon the subject of religion, disposed to be restless and talkative, violent, will fight any one who may as he supposes "cross" him, admitted May 1[st] 1853, died 9 June 1896, exhaustion.

465 **Miss Martha E. Mitchell**, pay patient, from Newton County, age about 19, single, supposed cause of insanity disordered health and religious excitement, duration 8 or 9 months, admitted May the 9 1853, address

Alexander Pharr, Esqr., Social Circle or Mrs. Julia A. Mitchell, Auburn, Ala., removed July 17<sup>th</sup> 1855.

466 **James B. Russell**, lunatic and epileptic from Muscogee County, age 30, duration 8 years, causes supposed bad health, violent, etc., for further history address Dr. Thos. P. Park, [?] Harris Co, and on all other occasions address Jas. M. Russell, Columbus, Geo., died May 26th 1855.

467 **Disey Perkins**, pauper lunatic and epileptic from Habersham County, age about 40, single, has been the subject of epilepsy since earliest childhood, insane for about 4 years, cause of insanity epilepsy suffering from partial paralysis, her habits filthy etc, admitted May 16 1853, died July 7th 1855.

468 **Mrs. Margaret Pevy**, pauper lunatic from Meriwether County, age about 31, widow, has one child seven years old, husband died in December 1850, has been insane about fourteen months, supposed cause loss of husband and one of her children, occupation ordinary household business, health failed about the time of her husband's death, and seemed to grow worse gradually until about fifteen or sixteen months back, when she experienced a very severe attack of typhoid fever, with some disease of the womb, since which time her mania has grown speedily worse, shows disposition to show acts of violence but rarely, usually much depressed, often noisy, admitted May 22nd 1855, discharged restored Apr 9 '56, address Robt Betts, Magadline, Meriwether County.

469 **Stephen Runnel**, pauper lunatic and epileptic from Dooly County, age about 28 years, single, farmer, duration of epilepsy about 15 or 16 years, supposed cause dropsy, paroxysms occur about once a week, for about fourteen months mind has seemed constantly disordered, is disposed to commit acts of violence towards others, at this time suffering from disordered bowels, general health feeble for 2 yrs past, never has been subjected to mechanical restraint until February last, admitted 25 May 1855, address Reuben Runnels, Hawkinsville, died July 16th 1855.

470 **Henrietta Jacobs**, pauper lunatic from Baker County, age about 25 years, single, insane for 5 years or more, ill treatment of her by different persons, her general health very good, admitted May 26 1855, died Jany 5th 1861.

471 **Mrs. Catora Parsons**, pauper lunatic from Floyd County, age about 40, duration of insanity five years or more, causes unknown, general health feeble, admitted May 27 185, died Sept 9th 1855.

472 **William C. Russel**, pay patient from Morgan County, Alabama, single, age about 27, duration 4 years, causes bad health and too close application, has been for a short time an inmate of the Nashville Institution, does not try to injure himself but has threatened the lives of those whose duty it has been to care for him, destructive to clothing, glass, etc., general health bad, is believed by his physician to have diseased liver, admitted 13 June 1855, removed Sept 28th 1855.

473 **Harvey C. Johnson**, pauper lunatic from Cherokee County, age about 37 years, married, farmer, duration 5 months, causes of insanity supposed "dropsy of Brain," fourteen years ago he became insane, was committed to lunatic asylum Columbia S.C., remained 6 months and was discharged restored, lived with and supported his family with an occasional return of disease, for which he was confined in county jail, his mind since first attack has been weak and his conduct at times strange and erratic, he is represented as being very violent, no suicidal tendencies, filthy in his habits, destructive to his clothing, window glass, etc., no particular delusions, [?] maniacal exhaustion 12 Nov 1855, admitted June 20 1855, address Harmon Halcom, Ball Ground P.O., Cherokee Co (written to), died Novr 12th 1855.

474 **Mary A[?] Adams**, pauper epileptic from Taylor County, admitted July 2 1855, died May 11th 1861.

475 **Walton H. Jones**, pay patient from Floyd County, age 40, married, farmer, duration of insanity one month, first symptoms manifested about 2 years ago, continuing with perfect intervals until one month ago when he became decidedly insane, causes continued intemperance, his prominent delusions are that he is immensely wealth, that all property belongs to him, also his disposition to purchase every article at a most unreasonable and extravagant price, he has had an attack of paralysis, he has at this time symptoms of the above, his habits are filthy and destructive to clothing, etc, admitted 14 July 1855, hereditary.

476 **Margaret Hennessy**, pauper lunatic form Chatham County, single, age 18 or 19, insane 4 or 5 mos, causes said to be disappointed affection and the failure to marry, no particular delusion, violent, destructive to clothing, etc., admitted [July] 15 1855, discharged Oct 1st 1855.

477 **Augustus Richards**, pay patient in part, from Talbot County, age 22, single, duration of insanity 5 years, became much worse a month ago, causes unknown, has attempted to destroy himself by taking laudanum, also shot a negro, admitted July 17 1855, eloped May 3rd 1856 much improved, returned Sept. 17th 1856, eloped Sept 1/58, readmitted Novr 1st 1858.

478 **Wm. J. Goode**, pauper epileptic from Franklin County, age 18 years, epileptic seizure commenced 2 years ago, causes self pollution, admitted Jul the 30 1855, died 23rd July 1876, epilepsy. Notified Ordinary.

479 **Elijah Smallwood**, pauper patient from Cobb County, age about 40, married, farmer, duration of insanity 12 months, causes unknown, also particular history, his general health bad, seems to be afflicted with paralysis, admitted July 31 1855, eloped Augt 15th 1855.

480 **Thomas Lambeth**, pauper lunatic and epileptic from Burke County, age about 61 years, duration 24 years, causes said to be religious excitement, delusions none particular, health bad, is paralytic, admitted August 2nd 1855, died Octr 15th 1855.

481   **R. Farwood**, pauper lunatic from Chatham County, 41 years old, Englishman, single, printer, history unknown, has been confined in jail in Savannah for 13 months, admitted Aug 5 1855, died 10th Jany 1870.

482   **George J. Spencer**, pauper lunatic from Chatham County, age 60, married, porter in bank for a number of years, duration of insanity 7 months, causes supposed diseased condition of spinal system and intemperance, has been incarcerated for 2 months, admitted Aug 5th 1855, died Aug 21/55.

483   **Flemming Childers**, pauper lunatic from Butts County, age 30 to 35, duration 2 months, causes intemperance, occupation keeping a grocery, general health good, sometime ago had acute inflammation of brain, on recovery returned to drink, had a 2nd attack followed by convulsions, since which mind has become impaired, violent, raving and sleepless (if likely do die, write to Miss L. A. Childers, Jackson), admitted Aug 4 1855, died Sept 12/55.

484   **Patrick Doyle**, pauper lunatic from Bibb County.

485   **Mary Ann Harrison**, pauper lunatic and epileptic from Franklin County, duration of insanity 6 years, of epilepsy 12 years, causes of insanity epilepsy, of epilepsy blow on head, not violent, health otherwise, admitted Aug 28, 1855.

486   **Greene M. Wiggins**, pauper lunatic from Greene County, age about 40 or 45, married, occupation carpenter, duration of insanity [blank], causes supposed seduction of his daughter connected with gross and excessive intemperance, is violent, noisy, destructive to his clothing etc, has no suicidal tendencies but will inflict injuries upon others, admitted Aug 31st 1855, discharged Novr. 15 1856.

487   **Cornelius Clarkson**, pauper epileptic and lunatic from Taylor County, age about 28, single, farmer, duration of insanity unknown, of epilepsy since infancy, cause of insanity epilepsy, disposed to fight, tries to kill his father by striking him with a rock, his habits are filthy, admitted Sept 12th 1855, died Dec 1st 1856.

487   **Thos. Blackstock**, pauper lunatic from Paulding County, age about 35, single, insanity has existed to some extent for ten years, causes unknown, general health usually good, farmer, has paroxysms of excitement in which he attempts acts of violence, throwing stones, health at this time not very good, admitted 13 Sept 1855.

488   **Elizabeth Cooper**, pauper idiot from Randolph County, single, age about 50, idiotic from birth, health good, destructive to clothing, etc., admitted Septr 21st 1855.

489   **Abram C. Martin**, pay patient from Meriwether County, age 33, first symptoms of insanity manifested several years ago, decidedly two or three years, causes supposed to be a sever attack of bilious fever, after recovery settled down in a hypochondriacal condition, gradually yielding

to insanity, has lucid moments, no particular elusions, at times violent and destructive, some hereditary tendency, admitted Oct 5 1855, Jan 1856 self pollution, the cause (exciting & continuing) of insanity.

489 **Salina Harden**, pay patient from Paulding County, age 21, duration 5 months, thinks her neighbors [?], causes unknown, generally mild but highly excitable if crossed, admitted Oct 5 1855, discharged Apl 26th 1856.

490 **Mary Busby**, idiot from Houston County, age 21 or 22, idiocy congenital, admitted October 9th 1855, if either she or Joseph Busby should die inform Mary Busby, Busbyville, Houston County.

491 **Archibald Thompson**, pauper patient from Screven County, age about 18 years, duration of lunacy 6 weeks, supposed cause religious excitement, tendency hereditary, very violent, tries to kill every thing that comes within his reach, destructive to his clothing, glass, &c., health good, admitted Oct 22nd 1855, address Seaborn Thompson, Sylvania P. Off. Screven County, discharged cured June 17 1856.

492 **George B. Bivel**, pauper lunatic from Taliaferro County, age [blank], married, occupation farmer, duration 7 or 8 years or more, cause unknown, not very violent, disposed to undress himself and to wander about, destructive to his clothing, filthy in his habits, has no suicidal tendency, has been for 18 months a lunatic of the asylum Columbia South Carolina, admitted Nov 2 1855.

493 **Daniel Obrian**, pauper lunatic from Muscogee County, age about 40 years, duration some three years, causes hard work and intemperance, disposed to strip himself, thinks it is his duty to preach, health not very good, disposition mild and quiet, is easily controlled, has been confined in jail for the last six months, admitted Nov 7th 1855, died 5th April 1870, dysentery.

494 **John P. Bon**, lunatic from McIntosh County, age upwards of 60 years, duration unknown, has been an inmate of asylum Columbia S.C., his [cause] unknown, health feeble, pauper, admitted Novr 8th 1855, eloped Sept 25 1858.

495 **Mary Porter**, pauper epileptic and idiot 16 or 17 years of age, idiocy result of epilepsy existent since infancy, admitted Nov 20 1855, died July 29 1857.

496 **Jacob Learer**, pauper lunatic from Wilkes County, single, age about 60 years, duration of insanity unknown, but supposed to have existed 40 years or more, cause unknown, has been blind for several years, health feeble, has done nothing for 10 or 12 years, admitted Nov 25 1855, died July 27 1856.

497 **Lucy Mooney**, pauper patient from Pickens County, age about 70, duration of disease 12 months, cause unknown, married, has had several children, present condition paralytic, at times very violent, will fight, does

not sleep well, has been treated but without effect, admitted Nov 30 1855, died July 20 1856.

498 **Edward H. Adams**, patient from Jasper County, age 33, farmer, married, first symptoms manifested 3 years ago, became decidedly insane 8 months back, causes unknown but supposed to be religious excitement, disease hereditary, his aunt uncle and sister are and have been insane, delusions witches riding him, will fight, will tear up his clothing, no suicidal tendency, temperate, admitted 5 Dec 1855, address Julia Adams, Gladesville, Jasper County, discharged June 13 1857.

499 **Robert M. Thompson**, pauper patient originally from Jasper County, sent to asylum from penitentiary, sentenced to 10 years imprisonment for assault with intent to murder, which took place more than two years ago, at that time doubtless to some extent insane, his conduct in penitentiary would fix upon the mind the [?], he there having made frequent attempts to kill without the slightest provocation, he is violent and dangerous, admitted December 7$^{th}$ 1855, died May 4$^{th}$ 1857.

500 **Robert Byrd**, pauper epileptic and lunatic from Lumpkin County, age 26, duration of insanity 7, of epilepsy since 10 years of age, doubtless with hereditary predisposition the cause of insanity, no prominent delusions, about once a month much worse and very violent, threatens to kill etc, health bad, [Drathen's cachectic], admitted December 13, 1855, Wm. Byrd, Crossville, Lumpkin Co., died Augt 25/56.

501 **Henry P. Duke**, pay patient and lunatic from Butts County, age 40, single, farmer, duration of insanity decided 2 months, first symptoms manifested 10 years ago, with occasional outbursts of mania, supposed to result from the death of a young female to whom he was engaged and very much attached, also the use of ardent spirits, has had epilepsy which doubtless exerted some agency, destructive, violent full of fight, &c, sleeps a good deal but in day time, admitted December 15 1855, address R. P. Duke, Jackson, Butts Co.

502 **Sarah Moody**, pauper lunatic and epileptic from Pike County, age about 20, duration of epilepsy and lunacy since 6 months of age, admitted January 1856, died Octr 16 1856.

503 **Samuel J. Milner**, pauper lunatic from Fayette County, age 45 or 50, farmer, single, duration 6 years, causes hereditary, committed to this institution in 1849, escaped, recommitted January 16 1856, died 17$^{th}$ June 1873.

504 **Bethina Farter**, pay patient from Greene County, age about 35, duration of insanity 4 years, causes and history to be furnished by husband, mother of 6 children, youngest 4 yrs of age, has been a patient in asylum Columbia S.C., insane 4 yrs, died March 26$^{th}$ 1867.

505 **Jno Bunyun Cook**, pay patient from Texas, discharged 23 Oct 1854, recommitted Feb 11 1856, causes masturbation, address Jesse M. Cook,

Dangerfield, Titus Co, Texas, address 7-25-1901, Mr. R. J. Cook, Winsboro, Wood Co, Tex, died 24 Aug 1903.

506 **Wm. Osborne**, pauper idiot and epileptic from Fayette County, age 28, congenital, admitted 20 Feb 1856, address Jonesboro, Fayette Co, Jno M. Osborne, died July 30th 1856.

507 **Frances McCormick**, pauper idiot from Spalding County, age 16 or 17, idiocy congenital and hereditary, admitted 21 Feb 1856, died March 3rd 1859, her system gave way from large number of fatty tumors.

508 **Moses W. Simmons**, pay patient from Taladega County, [Alabama], age 56, duration 3 years, 11 years ago became insane, taken to Kentucky asylum, was discharged cured, remained well until 3 yrs ago, became insane, becoming more quiet, noisy, violent, causes of first attack dyspepsia, no satisfactory cause assigned for last attack, noisy, violent, etc., admitted Feb 25 1856, discharged Oct 6th 1856.

509 **Columbia Pitts**, female, pauper, idiot from Troup County, admitted Mar 12 1856, died Sept 2nd 1857.

510 **Joseph Pharr**, pauper lunatic and epileptic from Gwinnett County, age about 24, married, has three children, duration of epilepsy 11 years, cause unknown, has for two years past had paroxysm at least once a week, sometimes more frequently, admitted Mar 14th 1856, died May 4 1857.

511 **Ezekiel Treadaway**, pauper patient from Floyd County, age 60, widower, has two sons, occupation farm laborer, duration of insanity very manifest for three years past but some indications of it have been observed for twenty years, general health at this time tolerably good, admitted Mar 28th 1856, eloped Nov 14 1856.

512 **Patsy Oliver**, Talbot County, lunatic, age about 45 years, widow, has no children, at present in tolerable health, generally peaceably disposed and industrious, supposed cause of insanity loss of property, duration five years, admitted March 29th 1856.

513 **Daniel Woodring**, pauper patient from Union County, age about 28, single, duration of insanity four years, cause overheat and [washing?] the river under such circumstances, admitted April 5th 1856, address Joseph Woodring, Shady Grove, Towns County, eloped Oct 16/57, retd. Decr 3/57.

514 **Decatur Crocket**, pauper patient from the penitentiary, insanity supervened after an attack of typhoid fever, duration about four months, admitted April 10 1856, has had two previous attacks of insanity, resulting from intemperance, eloped May 27 1858.

515 **James H. Anderson**, pay patient from Clarke County, married, has four children living, youngest about one year old, age about 34, duration of insanity about six years, cause loss of wife, ill heath and pecuniary embarrassment, has not been treated, has exhibited sometimes a tendency to cut his throat with a razor and has occasionally threatened to

commit acts of violence toward others but has never attempted either, generally restless at night, admitted April 15[th] 1856, discharged cured Jan 29 1857.

516 **Richard N. Westbrook**, pay patient form Houston County, age 46, youngest child 6 years old, duration ten or twelve years, occupation farmer, supposed cause a fall from a horse and the imposition of extraordinary business about the settlement of which he had much difficulty, never subjected to treatment, no disposition to suicide but occasionally disposed to commit acts of violence to others, admitted April 15 1856, 1862 May 22[nd] gone home on a visit, 186 Augt 5[th] returned to the institution.

516 **Mrs. Frances W. Welborn**, pay patient from Barber County, Alabama, age 32, married, has six children, youngest 3 years of age, hereditary tendency, duration of insanity and general history to be furnished by her husband, admitted April 18[th] 1856.

517 **George W. Mitchel**, pay patient epileptic and lunatic from Pensacola [Florida], age 47, duration of epilepsy about 35 years, his mind was discovered to be unsound at 2 or 3 years of age, at times disposed to be violent but is very feeble, admitted April 21 1846, died of epilepsy July 5[th] 1856.

518 **John C. Reed**, removed from the institution by his father contrary to the advice of the superintendent, though much improved, continued to do well at home for two months, working regularly, subsequently he became obstinate and ill natured and disposed to wander about the country, then made attempts to commit acts of violence and for two months past has been chained, admitted April 26 1856, died Jan 8 1857. See prior record.

519 **James Purbly**, pauper patient from the penitentiary, cause of insanity and duration unknown, was sentenced to the penitentiary at the March term of Superior Court of Coweta County, offence placing obstruction on the rail road, admitted May 9 1856, died Augt 2[nd] 1856.

520 **Alpheus McCrary**, pay patient from Talbot County, age about 21, single, duration of insanity uncertain, 7 or 8 years back he had an attack of fever, on recovery from which his mind appeared in some degree disordered, this state of things continued for about three months when he was considered entirely well, a recurrence of this state of things has taken place every year, those indications becoming every year more grave, and now his mind has been much [choored?] for two months during which time he has frequently threatened violence to his parents but has only attempted any thing of the kind, he has occasionally stripped himself, is usually quiet, general health feeble, seems dyspeptic, often complains of pain in his head, has contracted habits of self pollution, he frequently says there is a snake in his stomach, admitted May 15[th] 1851.

521 **Wm. Smith**, pauper idiot from Rabun County, age 31, condition congenital, admitted May 18[th] 1856.

522   **David Smith**, pauper idiot from Rabun County (brother of the above), age 35, congenital, admitted May 18. 56.

523   **Sarah Horn**, pauper lunatic from Jones County, age about 20, duration unknown, not dispose to injure herself as others, admitted May 20 1856, discharged Octr 1$^{st}$ 1857, readmitted, died 26 December 1904, senility.

524   **Catherine Moody**, pauper lunatic from Crawford County, age 32, widow, has 2 children, duration of insanity a few weeks, immediate cause of insanity unknown, the disease is hereditary, her mother and grandmother having been insane, not violent but troublesome, admitted May 27 1856, address Elisha P. Turner, Pine Level, Crawford Co, Ga.

525   **Mrs. Sarah M. Sheppard**, of Eufaula, Alabama, removed unimproved 24$^{th}$ Feby 1875.

526   **Mrs. Pamelia Holt**, pauper lunatic from Paulding County, age about 35, widow, with 4 children, husband died ten years back, duration of insanity more than ten years, the cause unknown, her general health at this time appears tolerably good, admitted July 13 1856.

527   **Miss Eliza McDonald**, partial pay patient from Cobb County, age about 30, duration of insanity 6 years, she improves at times, has been worse since the death of her father two years ago, cause of insanity unknown, no hereditary tendency, not particularly violent, admitted July 17$^{th}$ 1856, died Mar 29$^{th}$ 1861.

528   **Wm. M. Holt**, part pay patient from Savannah, age about 24, married, cause of insanity unknown, occupation engineer and machinist, duration of insanity about 4 months, has shown a disposition to commit acts of violence towards his mother and sister, has never tried to injure himself, received July 28 1856.

529   **S. M. Fambrough**, pauper lunatic from Oglethorpe County, age about 35, single, cause of insanity unknown, duration two years, general health tolerably good, has been near twelve months confined in jail, admitted July 29 1856.

530   **Miss Susan Goulding**, epileptic and lunatic from Burke County, age about 21, duration of epilepsy about 12 years, admitted July 30 1856, died Augt 22$^{nd}$ 1856.

531   **Miss Magadlene Wolf**, pauper idiot from Decatur County, condition congenital, age 37, admitted August 17 1856, died May 20 1858.

532   **George A. Boen**, pauper idiot from Clarke County, age [blank], health feeble, admitted August 6 1856.

533   **Jno. R. Alexander**, pay patient from Coweta County, age 33, single, for several years prior to the last past, post master, duration supposed to be three months, but probably much longer, cause believed to be ill health, has been subjected to very slight treatment, has not been confined or under mechanical restraint (that representation has proven altogether

incorrect), never attempts to commit acts of violence but often threatens, recd. Aug 9[th] 1856, discharged July 6 1857.

534 **John Bridges**, pauper patient from Greene County, idiot, age about 15 years, admitted August 13[th] 1856, died Dec 14/57 from a blow received from a patient.

535 **Thos. Perkins**, pauper idiot from Paulding County, age 26, deformed from birth, committed as an idiot but is said to have been of sound mind until eleven years of age, admitted August 19 1856, died Nov 14 1856.

536 **Miss Sarah Ann Oliver**, pauper idiot from Dougherty County, age [blank], deformed, admitted September 8[th] 1856, died July 29 1859.

537 **Mr. Nelson Hurley**, pauper lunatic of Gwinnett County, age about 25, single, farmer, cause of insanity unknown, duration two years or more, general health not good, is disposed to be destructive and also to commit acts of violence, admitted Sept 17 1856, address Joseph Googe, Lawrenceville, Ga, died 31[st] May 1871.

538 **Frances M. Edwards**, pay patient from Cherokee County, age about 31, married, has seven children, youngest now five months old, duration of insanity between two and three years, in January 54 she had mumps, very imperfectly developed though no manifest metastasis occurred, from that time certain persons alleged that they discovered something unusual in her deportment but nothing of the kind was noticed by her husband until a month later, the earliest indications of insanity observed by him were delusions in reference to departure from religious duties (she being a professor of religion and member of the Methodist church) and declarations that she had been bewitched and was worshipping the Devil, she was at that time in the 8[th] month of pregnancy, had smoked excessively for twelve or fourteen years prior to that time, has not used tobacco at all since, has sometimes been better but has never seemed entirely free from disorder of mind since Feb 54, general health has been good since that time, has now an infant in its 6[th] month, pregnancy and lactation have never seemed to exert any influence on the condition of her mind, has never been treated for insanity, has never been bled but once since in this condition, has never been subjected to mechanical restraint, it has been unsuccessfully attempted, has attempted violence toward her husband, for the first year appeared inordinately fond of her husband, since that time just the reverse and has grown constantly worse in that particular, about a year after the first manifestation of insanity her husband whipped her with a wagon whip, she seems to be at present in good general health, is neat and cleanly in her habits but occasionally destructive, admitted Oct 6[th] 1856, discharged cured Sept 15 1857.

539 **Archibald Pitts**, pauper patient from Coweta County, age 45 or more, married, has a wife from whom he is separated, has children, duration of insanity 4 or 5 years, is believed to have been formerly dissipated, but has not been recently, cause of insanity unknown, but supposed to be

disordered health, health feeble at present, has never been treated for insanity, has been confined to jail for three weeks, has exhibited a disposition to do mischief with fire, has fired several buildings and fences, received Oct 9ᵗʰ 1856, eloped April 14 1857.

540 **Elizabeth Warwick**, pauper lunatic from Lumpkin County, age 62, married, has 6 children, youngest 21 years of age, became insane forty years ago after the birth of her first child, remained insane six months, was not violent except when restrained, believed her father and mother in the sun, her husband removed to North Carolina where her parents resided, eight or ten years after the first attack became again insane at the birth of her fourth child, duration of second attack twelve months, was more violent than before, was confined to her room, after recovery continued entirely well until ten years ago when she was again attacked, imagines she is the Almighty that the Savior wishes to marry her, she became more troublesome two years ago, admitted Oct 21 1856.

541 **Maria E. Lowe**, pay patient from Chattooga County, age 36, married, has six children, youngest six years of age, last gestation occurred in 1852, child lived one month, after delivery suffered for a long time with phlegmasia dolens, since that time her health has been bad, has been nervous, disposed to melancholy unduly affected by loss of friends &c, but manifested no derangement of mind until last June, the attack occurred quite suddenly, supposed immediate cause misunderating [this word not clear] with her son in law, not violent but uses bad language, admitted Oct 25ᵗʰ 1856, address David C. R. Lowe, Summerville, Chattooga Co, Ga.

542 **Sarah Phillips**, pauper patient from Washington County, single, age about 25 or 30, duration of insanity two or three months, no satisfactory cause known, hereditary, her mother has been insane but has recovered, not violent nor destructive, is sometimes profane, a house was burned in her neighborhood sometime since which she says she fired, admitted Oct 30ᵗʰ 1856, discharged cured March 28 1858.

543 **Thos. J. Ingram**, pauper lunatic from Carroll County, age 25, single, occupation farmer, cause of insanity supposed to be result of a severe attack of typhoid fever which occurred four or five years ago, since that time his mind has been feeble, but he was not considered insane until two years ago, has no prominent delusions, usually melancholy but has exhibited no suicidal tendency, has shown no disposition to commit acts of violence until a short time since, no hereditary tendency, admitted Nov 10ᵗʰ 1856. If he should die while in the institution procure a burial case and write to A. J. Boggess or David Boling.

544 **Timothy C. Snelson**, pauper lunatic from Jackson County, age about 27, was brought to the institution in 1850, escaped Feb 1851 much improved, has however never entirely recovered, he has married since he left and has two children, the immediate cause of insanity unknown, but

hereditary, has a brother who has been in the asylum, admitted Nov 19 1856, eloped Dec 12 1858, since died in Alabama.

545 **Ellen A. Dent**, pay patient from Heard County, lunatic, age 39, single, duration of insanity 6 or 7 years, about twenty five years ago suffered from a severe attack of fever, since which time she has never enjoyed good health, nor has her mind been as active as before, six or seven years ago she was again attacked with fever complicated with uterine disease, from which she suffered for many months and during which she became decidedly insane, has never naturally improved, has occasional paroxysms of excitement but is usually quiet, has lived for six or seven years in a small house in her father's yard (generally alone) remaining almost all of the time in the house from choice admitted Nov 22 1856.

546 **Miss Annie Budd**, partial pay patient from Baldwin County, epileptic, duration of epilepsy 2 years, mind does not seem affected, admitted Dec 1$^{st}$ 1856.

547 **Wm. J. Murphy**, pauper idiot from Houston County, age 35 years, admitted Decr 11$^{th}$ 1856, died of pneumonia and dysentery April 4$^{th}$ 1858.

548 **James Boyd**, pauper lunatic committed from Meriwether County, is supposed to be a resident of Fayette County, nothing is known of his history, he had been wandering about Greenville for a short time before his commitment, admitted Dec 12$^{th}$ 1856.

549 **W. J. D. Smiley**, pay patient from [blank] County, age [blank], duration of insanity [blank] years, was committed to the asylum in 185[blank], effected his escape two or three times, was at one time in the Worcester Asylum, is sometimes violent, has attempted suicide, health at this time only tolerably good, admitted December 20 1856, removed by friends Jan 15 1858, died Oct 12/62.

550 **Mrs. McClesky**, pay patient from [blank], age [blank], duration of insanity [blank] years, history of her case furnished superintendant by her brother, admitted December 23$^{rd}$ 1856.

551 **Mrs. Caroline Deason**, pauper patient from Wilkinson County, has 3 children, duration of insanity about 4 years, has been much worse for six months, is at this time in an excited state, health bad, admitted December 26 1856, dischd Feby 28 1857, readmitted, discharged March 21$^{st}$ 1862.

552 **Samuel T. Burns**, patient from Wilkes County, history of the case not received, admitted December 26 1856, discharged cured April 5$^{th}$ 1858.

553 **Sarah McLeod**, pauper patient from [blank] County, epileptic, duration of epilepsy [blank] years, admitted December 31 1856, died April 16 1858.

554 **Susan Wadkins**, pauper lunatic from DeKalb County, single, age 33, was insane 15 years ago, has been much better at times, became worse 15 months since, has not improved since that time, has been confined to jail

for several months, cause supposed to be uterine derangement, admitted January 7 1857, discharged cured July 24 1859.

555 **Mr. W. A. Woodburn**, pay patient from Decatur County, age 20, single, has been in ill health for two years past and under the treatment of a physician, but no indication of insanity until six or eight months ago, cause of ill health and insanity supposed to be masturbation, admitted January 8[th] 1857.

556 **Miss Anna L. Keaton**, pauper lunatic from Carroll County, history of the case unknown, she is violent and destructive, admitted Jan 8[th] 1857, died July 25 1857.

557 **James Davis**, pay patient of Morgan County, age 17, duration of insanity certainly ten days, probably for one year, has had no severe attack of illness nor any manifestation of indisposition sufficient to attract attention, the first marked manifestation of derangement of mind was a disposition to converse in public on religion and to pray at unseemly times and places, he then occasionally attempted to commit acts of violence toward his brother in law and other near friends but showed no hostility toward strangers, is not disposed to suicide, is not destructive, is disposed to be filthy, has defecated in his clothing, has been subjected to the confinement of a straight jacket for three or four days, was under medical treatment, was bled purged &c but without benefit, rested not more than a few minutes for ten past until since three o'clock yesterday since which time he has slept ten or twelve hours, admitted Feb 15[th] 1857, discharged cured Oct 1[st] 1857.

558 **Duke Myers**, pauper patient from Sumter County, age about 50, married, has five children, member of the Methodist church, was never remarkably intelligent, has borne good character for morality &c, some of his friends think they have perceived a change in his conduct for two years, but nothing of the kind has been observed by his family until four months since, about which time his family were accused of setting fire to fencing on a neighboring plantation which gave rise to a difficulty in the church that caused him a great deal of anxiety, refuses to answer questions or to converse, is generally peaceable and quiet, has attempted suicide by trying to cut a tree down on himself, afterwards begged his wife to remove everything from him with which he could harm himself, is not destructive, health only tolerable, admitted Feb 28[th] 1857, address C. A. Thompson, Americus, Ga., died Oct 8 1857.

559 **Titus A. Davis**, pauper lunatic from Baldwin County, age about [blank], single, was sentenced to the penitentiary from Decatur County for horse stealing, was discharged from prison last fall, supposed at that time by many to be laboring under insanity, has remained about Milledgeville ever since, sleeping in the open air during the winter and dependent upon the charity of the community for food, admitted March 14[th] 1857, died 29 Aug 1897, exhaustive mania.

560   **Henry J. Miller**, pauper patient from Ware County, age 65, duration of insanity first indications noticed by his family 9 or 10 months ago, at which time he began to neglect his business (having been previously very attentive to business), he also became extremely taciturn and indifferent to every thing around him, has never attempted to commit any act of violence until several weeks since when he attempted to shoot his son and struck him with a stick, cause unknown, received a severe blow on the heat from a cotton bale some years ago but has shown no symptoms of insanity noticeable to the family until August last, admitted April 8$^{th}$ 1857, died May 21$^{st}$ 1862.

561   **Miss Sarah Chandler**, from Gilmer County, pauper epileptic and lunatic, age 21, duration 5 years, cause supposed to be loss of her parents, admitted April 14$^{th}$ 1857.

562   **James Denton**, pay patient from Bibb County, married, has a wife and one child, age 44, duration of insanity 9 years or more, was attacked with a convulsion while in apparent health, ever since which his mind has been more or less disordered, the convulsions have recurred at uncertain intervals since but has had none for a year past, is now in a state of partial paralysis, about one a month has a paroxysm of excitement in which he will strike persons about him, bite and scratch himself, &c, is disposed to do mischief with fire, admitted April 17 1857, died Nov 5 1857.

563   **Orsborn R. Johnson**, pay patient form Gordon County, age about 42 years, has a wife and 4 children, duration of insanity about 20 months, cause unknown unless an injury of the head received 12 years previously, has suicidal tendencies, is quiet and orderly, rests well, admitted April 26 1857, disch June 27 1857.

564   **Wm. M. Warwick**, pauper patient from Lumpkin County, age 22 years, single, has been insane it is believed nearly all his life, cause hereditary, usually quiet but sometimes irritable and disposed to commit acts of violence toward his family, has not attempted any thing of the sort toward others, is cowardly and easily influenced to do what he is directed, admitted May 1$^{st}$ 1857, eloped Sept 3$^{rd}$ 1858, eloped June 5/57, returned Sept 24/57, eloped Oct 15 1857.

565   **Jonathan Melton**, pauper patient from Clarke County, lunatic and epileptic, age about 29 years, duration of epilepsy from 2 years of age, experienced exemption from convulsions from 7 to 14 years of age when they recurred and have continued ever since, now has a convulsion about once a week, his mind has appeared permanently disordered for about 7 years, usually quiet never dispose to acts of violence unless irritated, received May 7 1857, address Mrs. Sarah Melton, Athens, Ga.

567   **John H. Moore**, pay patient, lunatic and epileptic of Baldwin County, age about 32 years, single, duration of epilepsy about 30 years, supposed cause malformation of skull, health generally good, usually quiet but sometimes irritable, has convulsions very frequently, sometimes occurring

three or more times during the day and night, admitted May 11, 1857, died of chronic diarrhea May 6 1858.

568    **Hiram Addcock**, pauper lunatic from Cobb County, age about 45 years, has been married, it is not known whether his wife is living, has no children, duration of insanity seven years or more, cause unknown, sometimes excited and destructive, has never shown suicidal tendencies and rarely disposed to commit acts of violence towards others, admitted June 5 1857, eloped Mar 29/61.

569    **Miss Mahulda Coward**, pauper lunatic from Pickens County, age about 32 years, single, has one child about 9 years old, cause of insanity unknown, has always been regarded as weak minded, has been decidedly insane for some weeks only, has been subjected to mechanical restraint, admitted June 6th 1857, address P. C. Coward, Jasper, Pickens Co., Ga., discharged cured Oct 1st 1857.

570    **Mrs. Mary Ann Lindsay**, pay patient from Macon, married, has five children, youngest 3 months of age, has been in the asylum before, see page 9th, duration of insanity five years, admitted Jan 6th 1857, discharged cured April 22nd 1859.

571    **Seaborn Reynolds**, pauper lunatic from Floyd County, age 18 years, single, duration of insanity near a year, mind has been feeble all his life, cause unknown, his mother was insane once for a short time, two months back he was very violent and troublesome, has been under medical treatment, purged freely and bled twice, admitted July 18 1857, discharged cured Oct 1st 1857.

572    **Mrs. Mary S. Jones**, pay patient from Whitfield County, age 34 years, was married eight years ago, seventeen months after marriage had a child, has never been pregnant since, no indication of derangement of mind was exhibited until last March, general health has been good, her menstrual function seemed to be in a natural state until recently, so far as known, has complained for three or four months past of peculiar pains in her head, is generally restless during the latter part of the night and appears worse every morning, has attempted suicide in different ways, in the last instance cut her throat with a razor, admitted June 20 1857, died Jan 15 1858, committed suicide by hanging.

573    **Jas. L. Hinton**, pay patient from Meriwether County, single, age 25 years, first indications of insanity noticed about a year ago, manifested by fickleness and restlessness, removed west with his property twice or three times and returned in as many months, is a member of the Baptist church, no hereditary tendency known, cause of insanity said to be disappointment in love, health has been generally good, has attempted no act of violence, has threatened the life of a gentleman in his neighborhood whose daughter it is said he loves, admitted June 27 1857.

574    **Mrs. Abigail Hardee**, pauper patient from Wilkinson County, age 43 years, has been a widow 13 years, has one child 15 years of age, duration

of insanity 2 years, perhaps longer, has had a good deal of sickness, had a severe attack of typhoid fever about 2 years ago, lost her father with whom she resided about the same time, has suffered from menstrual derangement for some years, the discharge has usually been slight, missed at the last period altogether, admitted June 29 1857, address Mrs. Christian McLeod, guardian, discharged Oct 1st 1857, returned Jan 30 1858.

575 **Peter Clark**, pauper patient from Burke County, an Irishman, age about 21 years, very little known of him, has been in Burke only a few weeks, seems to be humourous and mischievous, but not dangerous or violent, admitted July 2nd 1857, discharged Oct 1st 1857.

576 **Peter Dickson**, pauper patient from Muscogee County, an Irishman, age [blank], very little is known of his history, came to Muscogee County about 10 months ago, was laboring under insanity at that, is at times much better than at others, nothing is known of his family or friends, admitted July 3d 1857.

577 **Miss Samantha Ham**, pauper lunatic and epileptic from Twiggs County, age about 22 years, single, cause supposed menstrual derangement, duration of disease two years, general health bad for three or four years previously, now has convulsions twice a week or more frequently, has recently attempted to cut her throat and to drown herself, was formerly destructive, has not been so this year, has been under treatment for epilepsy, for three years, received July 20 1857, discharged cured June 15 1859.

578 **Mrs. Eliza Ann Moore**, pauper lunatic from Fayette County, age about 40 years, married, has had eleven children, has seven living, duration of insanity supposed two or three months, cause believed to be ill treatment by her husband and his bad conduct generally, she was deranged some two years back but was supposed to have recovered, general health only tolerable, received July 21st 1857, address Sandford W. Moore, Rough & Ready, removed 17th July 1877, improved.

579 **Mrs. Sarah J. Harris**, pay patient from Meriwether County, age 36 years, widow, has had five children, has two living, has resided for several years in Montgomery, Ala., but a native of Augusta, Geo., duration of insanity at this time supposed to be only five or six weeks, has been insane twice before, first attack eight years back, last three years back, cause not well understood, general health tolerably good, received July 28 '57, died 14th Sept 1878, general debility, notified.

580 **James S. Gibson**, pay patient from Chatham County, born in Savannah, age 24 years, single, duration of insanity uncertain, prominent and decided indications only for three months past, cause disordered health, from which he has suffered all his life, but as his health improved, which it has done recently to some extent, his mind has seemed to grow worse, has shown a disposition to wander off from home, his bowels generally loose, has suffered constantly for some months past with uneasiness in his head,

never disposed to commit acts of violence, appetite rather excessive, generally rests well at night, will be sure to run away if he gets an opportunity, received Aug 4<sup>th</sup> 1857, in case of Gibson [*sic* – death], address his guardn. J. K. Munnerly in Savannah Geo., died Oct 26 1858.

581   **Mrs. Sarah C. Girtman**, pay patient from Sumter County, age about 34 years, widow with six children living, has lost two, youngest child about 2 years old, duration of insanity about 34 months back, her husband was killed by a tree falling upon him, since which time her mind has appeared in some degree affected, but no very palpable manifestations of such a state occurred until three or four weeks back, is often excited, noisy, and destructive, has not attempted any serious act of violence, has been treated to some extent, been blistered and taken cathartic, head shaved &c., but not bled, disinclined to eat and does not sleep well, decided hereditary tendency in the family, one of her sisters died at the asylum in Columbia, S.C., received Aug 4 '57, address Mr. J. W. C. Horne, her brother, at Danville, Sumter Co., Geo., if she should die, her remains are to be sent home, died 17<sup>th</sup> July 1877, maniacal exhaustion, notified.

582   **Mr. James H. Yancey**, pauper patient from Forsyth County, lunatic and epileptic, age about 26 years, duration of disease unknown, cause supposed intemperance, ordinarily quiet unless drinking, then very violent and dangerous, received Aug 27 '57.

583   **Esekiel Butler**, partial pay patient from Dooly County, duration an indefinite period, worse for a year past, cause unknown, has attempted suicide by trying to cut his throat with his pocket knife, has tried to cut his tongue out with shears, has been very violent, has knocked down several persons, has been chained for some time, was much better in the spring but has been getting worse for some time, age 51 years, health feeble, admitted Sept 7 1857, address David T. Fo[?] or John Butler, Vienna, Dooly Co, Ga., discharged Jan 7 1858, returned of his own accord in May, discharged 30<sup>th</sup> November 1866.

584   **Chas. W. Nixon**, pauper patient from Carroll County, age about 50 years, duration of insanity said to be about one year, was insane a short time about ten years ago, suffered very much about a year ago from furuncles or carbuncles, was confined to the house for some months during which time he became insane, has suffered with head ache and somewhat from dyspepsia, has never used any violence toward himself or toward others, does not sleep well, is exceedingly noisy, especially at night, is averse to leaving the house, admitted Sept 8 1857, address Mrs. Mary Nixon, Laurehill, Carroll Co, Ga., removed Dec 11 1858.

585   **Wm. D. Gilmore**, pauper patient from Lee County, age about 19 years, health bad, duration of insanity said ix months, cause unknown, probably onanism, has once or twice attempted acts of violence, believes he has been poisoned by a Dr. Green of Lee County, avoids society, shuts himself in his room, admitted Sept 16 1857, address [blank], died Decr. 30<sup>th</sup> 1860.

586 **Allen Pucket**, pay patient from Coweta County, age 55 to 60 years, single, has kept a liquor shop for some years, has been very intemperate which is the cause of his insanity, has had delirium tremens, has been insane for six or eight months, is sometimes excited and disposed to violence but not often, has burnt some houses in his vicinity and may be properly watched, admitted September 18th 1857, died 27th July 1872, paralysis.

587 **Wm. N. Hill**, pay patient from Cobb County, age about 45 years, a resident of Fayette County, committed from Cobb, occupation Farmer, is a widower, has three children, duration of insanity unknown, history of the case cannot be obtained, admitted Oct 1857, died December 4th 1857.

588 **Cornelia Snellings**, epileptic from Jones County, age [blank] years, duration of epilepsy six years, convulsions generally occur at night, admitted October 24 1857, died 17th May 1870, epilepsy.

589 **J. C. Pollard**, pauper patient from Paulding County, occupation lawyer and teacher, married, has one child, married in Paulding, duration of insanity known to be 15 or 18 months, has been somewhat dissipated, admitted Oct 26 [blank - 1857], address [blank].

590 **Henry Hirshler**, German, occupation baker, period of insanity unknown, probably but a short time, continued to work at his trade until about two months ago, since that time has been confined in jail, is very destructive to his clothing but has not been violent, has shown no suicidal tendency, admitted October 27 1857, died Nov 23 1858.

591 **Mrs. Celestia Johnson**, partial pay patient from Troup County, age 22 years, widow, has three children, was married at 12 years of age, lost her husband six months before the birth of her youngest child, duration of insanity about 3 years, became insane at the birth of her last child, has been violent and destructive, is extremely noisy, has been kept tied for about two years, admitted Oct 28th 1857, address Hiram Dennis, Long Cane, Troup County, Ga., removed Dec 13 1858.

592 **Wm. M. Forster**, pauper patient from Floyd County, married, has three children, has been very dissipated, has not drank recently, was in the Creek, Florida, and Mexican wars, was sane previous to going to Mexico except when under the influence of ardent spirits at which times he was very violent, he returned from Mexico laboring under Mexican diarrhea and showed some symptoms of insanity then, was dissipated then, the insanity became much more marked two years ago, probably had an attack of manic[*illeg.*], he has an Aunt who has suffered from insanity, has been blind 3 years, has been operated on for cataract several times without permanent benefit, admitted Nov 5th 1857, address R. S. Forster, Rome, Ga.

593 **Mrs. Mary Walker**, pauper patient from Morgan County, cause unknown but probably the result of an unhappy marriage, has been married 12 or 14 years, has four children, has suicidal tendencies, duration of insanity

unknown, certainly six months, probably longer, admitted Nov 12th 1857, address John W. Porter, Madison, Ga., discharged cured Oct 1st 1858.

594 **Elias Lee**, Calhoun County, age 35 years, married, has 3 children, has been twice before in the institution, was discharged cured April 14th 1855, remained well until 18 months back, relapsed, supposed to have resulted from intemperance, about a year ago became lame, has been unable to walk since, caused by rheumatism, general health not good, admitted Nov 27 1857, died 28th Nov 1878, notified.

595 **Miss Dolly Ann Davis**, pauper lunatic from Marion County, age 33 years, unmarried, duration of insanity 6 years, has been kept chained 2 years, has been several times severely whipped by her father, very destructive, to some extent the subject of pyromania, cause of insanity not positively known, not hereditary was disappointed in love some years ago, suffered for some time from retention of menses, has also suffered from some disease of urinary organs, usually careless and filthy in her habits, admitted Nov 27 1857, address Francis Davis, Buena Vista, Ga., died June 6/62.

596 **Mr. Ellis M. Waller**, pauper lunatic from Hancock County, age about [blank] years, duration of insanity not positively known, probably 18 months, cause supposed to be intemperance, is married, has several children, admitted Nov 28 1857, died 17th June 1882.

597 **John Evans**, pay patient, from Morgan County, age 19 years, single, is an orphan, duration of insanity, was not known to be insane more than a month, cause of insanity unknown, has dissipated to some extent but not recently, has been exceedingly anxious to get his property into his own hands, has not been able to do it, has been very much worried on that account, admitted December 2nd 1857, address C. Camble, Madison.

598 **James T. Wiley**, pauper lunatic from Cobb County, age 61 years, duration of insanity [blank], history of the case unknown, admitted December 3d 1857, died Mar 22nd 1861.

599 **James M. Sorrells**, pay patient from Walton County, age 22 years, single, duration of insanity 3 years, cause unknown, has dissipated some little, at the time the first symptoms were first notice was in apparent health, no hereditary tendency, is destructive and sometimes very violent, is the subject of sudden and violent impulses at which times he would kill his best friends, admitted December 3 1857, died May 15, 1866.

600 **Mrs. Susannah Springer**, pauper patient from Troup County, married, has five children, youngest two years old, age about 35 years, duration of insanity 12 years, has better sometimes for a month or two, cause hereditary predisposition, her father was insane 10 years, has been well 20 years, has a brother rather idiotic, has a sister who is insane in Alabama, probable immediate cause harsh treatment of her husband who is dissipated and worthless, he deserted her a short time ago taking the children with him, she wandered in the woods for two days, she is

destructive but not very violent, admitted December 3d 1857, address [blank] Loyd, LaGrange., Ga.

601 **James B. Warren**, pauper patient from Jackson County, age 20 years, single, occupation farmer, duration said to be only 6 months, not very violent nor destructive, cause unknown, admitted December 7[th] 1857, address Wm. Warren, Jefferson, Jackson Co., died of dysentery of a very malignant form, May 14[th] 1858.

602 **Mrs. Margaret J. Booker**, pauper patient from Telfair County, age 22 years, duration first symptoms of insanity noticed last May, no hereditary tendency, has one child 3 years old, lost a child last January, 2 days old, her health has been bad ever since, has never menstruated since the birth of her last child, has been troubled with prolopsus uteri, has strong suicidal tendencies, set herself on fire, has tried to get knives, ropes, etc., for the purpose of self destruction, has several times quit eating for two or three days, at this time has eaten nothing for seven days, has not spoken for two weeks, has refused to walk or stand for several days, admitted December 7[th] 1857, address Chas. Booker, Lumber City, Ga., died May 20 1858.

603 **Mrs. Mary E. Carlton**, pauper patient from Walton County, age 25 years, single, supposed cause of insanity ill health, six or seven years back had erysipelas, had several attacks previously, was bled freely when the eruption suddenly disappeared, since which time her health has not been good and occasionally she has been unnaturally fretful and excitable, has been sick only two or three times and then not seriously, her mind seemed worse during those attacks, has shown some disposition to suicide by knocking her head against the wall, is disposed to commit acts of violence, has attempted to kill her mother, will burn everything she can lay hands on, received Dec 15 1857, died 13[th] June 1876, Ordinary [judge] notified.

604 **Miss Mary Davenport**, pauper idiot from Marion County, age 30 years, cause of idiocy supposed to be injury from a fall which her mother received during her pregnancy, her father and mother are related to each other, admitted Dec 18[th] 1857, address Wm. A. Bell, Buennavister [Buena Vista], Marion County, Ga, died June 23/60.

605 **Mrs. Jenette Barley**, pauper lunatic from Gordon County, age about 50 years, married, duration of insanity three and a half years, cause unknown, is not now disposed to injure herself but attempts violence toward others, is often very much excited and noisy, has been confined only when excited, youngest child thirteen years old, admitted Decr. 24[th] 1857.

606 **Sofronia Baily**, pauper idiot, seemed as intelligent as any other child of her parents until three years of age when she experienced a severe attack of illness, after which she did not speak for three years, since then she has

spoken freely and enjoyed fine health, she is now about seventeen years of age, admitted Decr 24 1857, died 25 Feby 1918, meumonia [pneumonia].

607 **E. D. Johns**, pay patient from Polk County, age 47 years, married, duration of insanity one month, nineteen years ago was insane for two months, he then lived in Virginia, it is by no means certain that his mind has been entirely sound since his previous insanity, cause supposed to be a difficulty with his minister, he being a Methodist, had pneumonia in the spring, has shown no suicidal disposition but is disposed to commit acts of violence toward others and to do mischief with fire, general health is rather feeble, admitted Decr 24th 1857, discharged cured Feb 2nd 1858.

608 **Thos. D. Watson**, pauper lunatic from Lee County, age 27 years, single, duration of insanity about 20 years, cause supposed hereditation, is usually very quiet, sometimes excited somewhat, never attempted violence toward himself or others except by striking them with his hand when excited, health generally good, at present in a state of dementia, health feeble, appetite good but does not rest well, has never been treated, has never been confined, is sometimes disposed to ramble off, received Decr. 28 1857, address Thos. D. Watson, Albany, Ga.

609 **Wm. Poppell**, pauper lunatic from Liberty County, age 35 years, married, has one child, duration of insanity two years or thereabout, supposed cause intemperance and loss of money, has never been treated, has shown no suicidal tendency, not destructive, seldom excited and has never attempted violence toward other persons, received Jan 10 1858.

610 **James B. Parker**, pauper patient from Tattnall County, age 25 years, was the subject of epilepsy when an infant but recovered from it and was free from the disease until 14 years of age, it has continued ever since, admitted Jan 15 1858, address L. A. H. Tippens, Bull Creek, Tattnall Co., died Nov 15/61.

611 **William Dorris**, pauper idiot from Cherokee County, age about 60 years, is a widower, has no children, his father and mother were own cousins, admitted Jan 18, 1858, died March 30/61.

612 **Margaret Dorris**, pauper idiot from Cherokee County, age over 50 years, is a sister of William, admitted Jan 18 1858.

613 **Jincy Carpenter**, pauper epileptic from Cherokee County, age about 40 years, a widow, has had epilepsy from childhood, admitted Jan 18 1858.

614 **Eliza A. Lowry**, pauper lunatic from Cherokee County, single, age about 20 years, duration of insanity about three years, had an attack of typhoid fever, was found to be insane during her recovery, menstruation has been irregular ever since, occurring at longer intervals than natural, is violent and destructive, has been tied at times to prevent her doing mischief, has never been treated for insanity, has never attempted violence toward herself, admitted Jan 18 1858, address Henry Lowry, Cherokee Co, Ga., died May 19th 1862.

615   **Joseph Phelps**, pay patient from Florida, married, age about 40 or 45 years, duration of insanity unknown, whole history unknown, he came to Santa Rosa County, Florida, three years ago and was then insane, received January 22 1858. ($250)

616   **William Wier**, pauper patient from Newton County, age [blank] years, duration of insanity [blank].

617   **Mrs. Mary A. Hubbard**, pay patient from Richmond County, was discharged from the institution Oct 1ˢᵗ 1856, for former history see page 10, admitted Jan 26, 1858.

618   **Mrs. Civility Roberts**, pauper patient from Screven County, age about 45 years, widow, has three children, all grown, duration of insanity about 17 years, cause supposed to be intemperance of her husband, became insane during recovery from a long attack of illness, is violent and destructive at times, admitted Jan 28 1858.

619   **George Walker**, pay patient from Jackson County, Alabama, age about 40 years, widower, has three children living, duration of insanity about ten years, supposed cause injury of head in youth and intemperate habits, about ten years ago he had a dispute with his brother, about the lines of their land, and, in a state of intoxication attacked and killed him with a knife, was then confined in jail and remained in jail until last April when under conviction of insanity the judge released him on bail, was out only six weeks when being intoxicated he attempted to shoot his brother in law and was returned to jail, has attempted acts of violence only when intoxicated, except once when he had a fight with a prisoner who occupied the same room with him while in jail, has never attempted suicide, is indifferent to personal neatness but not destructive, has never been subjected to any treatment, has a brother who is believed to be insane, received Jan 29 1858, died Octr 31ˢᵗ 1862. ($250)

620   **Mrs. Abigail Hardee**, pauper patient from Wilkinson County, second admission, see page 9, received Jan 30 1858, died Feby 14ᵗʰ 1861.

621   **Mrs. Mary E. Faver**, pay patient from Meriwether County, age 28 years, is married, has three children, youngest nine years old, duration of insanity eight years, became better for a few weeks, a month or two after she was first attacked, cause unknown, health not good, menstrual function very much disordered, has been violent but is not at all so now, has attempted suicide several times, once by strangulation with a handkerchief, on one occasion she dressed herself in white, had a tub of warm water carried to her room and prepared to destroy herself with a knife, she has made no such attempt for years, seems at this time but little removed from a state of dementia, received Jan 30 1858.

622   **Eugene M. Gavan**, partial pay patient from Savannah, age about 20 years, occupation printer, second admission, see page 25, was discharged cured, may 1855, remained well until a few weeks since, cause of recent attack supposed to be novel reading, together with some pecuniary

difficulties, is noisy, violent and restless, will dance for hours, has recently been confined to jail, received Jan 30 1858, discharged cured Sept 1$^{st}$ 1858. (pay patient for six months)

623    **Miss Bridget Downey**, pauper lunatic from Chatham County, age [blank] years, single, duration of insanity two years or more, cause unknown, has been under treatment at the city hospital of Savannah for two years, received Feb 3$^{rd}$ 1858, died 27$^{th}$ Nov 1872.

624    **Mrs. Elizabeth Holden**, patient from Cass County, to pay five dollars per annum, age about 40 years, married, has four children, youngest child two years old, duration of insanity uncertain, supposed to be recent, supposed cause sudden and violent death of one of her children two years ago, is supposed to commit acts of violence upon herself and others, is very destructive and sometimes noisy, has been subjected frequently to personal restraint, strong hereditary predisposition, was insane 20 years ago,  a sister of hers hung herself and a brother Mr. John D. Hatch died in this institution, received Feb 3$^{rd}$ 1858, discharged on account of pregnancy, Mar 17/[*illeg.* 58? 66?].

625    **Henry Falkner**, patient from Hall County, married, occupation farmer, age 24 years, duration of insanity less than one year, no palpable evidence of insanity until last October at which time he started to Texas with his family, acted singularly while loading his but his conduct attracted no special attention, went two days journey, was found to be insane, said he was in Texas, left the camp and went hunting, preached, sometimes very violent and destructive, is disposed to do mischief with fire, was brought to the asylum in chains, has been kept chained most of the time since October, no special cause known, strong hereditary predisposition, has had two aunts, sisters of his father, who have been insane, his mother has also been insane, all recovered, his general health is at this time very good, received Feb 4 1858, discharged cured March 30 1858.

626    **Andrew J. Camp**, pauper lunatic and epileptic from DeKalb County, age about 20 years, single, duration of insanity about 4 years, of epilepsy 8 years, supposed hereditary predisposition, mother had epilepsy and other members of the family two generations were insane, epileptic convulsions occur frequently generally every day, never one interval longer than one week, is sometimes violent and disposed to assault persons about him, not destructive to clothing or bedding, will endeavor to run off, has no suicidal tendencies, received Feb 23d 1858, died Oct 19$^{th}$ 1859.

627    **Calvin Wolf**, pauper lunatic from Effingham County, age about 36 years, married, has a wife and seven children, farmer and timber cutter, duration of insanity about three years, cause supposed to be severe attack of illness, attended with abscesses in his ears, generally quiet but sometimes violent, threatens to assault persons about him, has never committed an act of violence, not at all destructive, has shown no suicidal tendency, has been treated by several physicians, received February 23d 1858, address Mrs. Sabina Wolf, Egypt, Effingham County.

628 **James G. Atkinson**, pauper lunatic from Fulton County, age 44 years, occupation laborer, duration of insanity about 8 years, about a year after becoming insane became much better and continued better until recently, but never entirely recovered, became much worse a short time since, but followed his occupation as laborer until last Friday, has suicidal tendencies, is sometimes rather violent, health poor, mind has never been particularly bright, supposed cause had a fall about a year previous to his insanity, by which it was thought his head may have been injured, about the inception of the disease suffered very much from a carbuncle between his shoulders, remote cause hereditation, his father has been insane several years, admitted March 6 1858, address John Atkinson, Atlanta, Ga., discharged [Sept?] 25 1859.

629 **Irwin Kirkland**, pauper lunatic from Emanuel County, age 42 years, a native of the county, married, occupation farmer, member of the Baptist church, the first indications of insanity were observed a year ago, perhaps longer, suppose cause pecuniary embarrassment, the first indications were a disposition to ramble off without any definite design, at which he travelled to considerable distances from home on foot, is believed to have lucid intervals, has never attempted to injure himself, has threatened violence to others but never attempted, has been confined to jail for 25 days, is never noisy or violent, is not destructive, is not filthy in his habits, he seems to have remained in about the same condition or the past six months, speaks of killing his children, says he is obliged to do so before he dies, and offer them up in sacrifice to God, nothing is known of his hereditary predisposition, has used tobacco to excess, admitted March 15 1858, address Mrs. Kirkland, Midville, Ga., eloped June 9 1858.

630 **Hugh G. Armstrong**, pauper epileptic from Walker County, age about 17 years, born in South Carolina but has lived in Walker Co. since he was a small boy, single, occupation farmer, first convulsion occurred when he was about five years old, had an attack of fever and about a month after he got up was attacked with convulsions, is attacked often at night, is sometimes to commit acts of violence toward others, is attacked often at night, is [*unclear*] not destructive, received March 16 1858, died August 24 1858.

631 **Dr. Francis C. Coleman**, pauper lunatic from Houston County, age about 27 years, for the past five or six years has had no regular employment, he studied medicine, attended lectures in Philadelphia and in 1854 settled in the practice in Lee County, remained there only about three months, he then went to Texas where he again practiced medicine, in October last he was brought back to Houston County in consequence of derangement of mind, is not a professor of religion, habits bad for ten years past, being intemperate and in the practice of other excesses, has drunk liquor to excess for 8 or 10 years, has drunk but little for 4 or 5 months, general health has been usual good, his mind seems mainly occupied by the idea that he has been involved in serious difficulty and is constantly anticipating punishment for some act of violence which he has

committed, no important change in his condition since his return from Texas, has never been treated, received March 17, 1858, eloped Jany 28/62, returned Feby 9/62, eloped June 26/62.

632   **Reuben Cobb**, pauper patient from Union [County], age about 25 years, single, is a member of the Methodist church, formerly he was a school teacher, his health having become impaired quit teaching and went to North Carolina for the purpose of mining, very little is known of his condition while there, remained in North Carolina one year, came home two years ago in a state of mental derangement, traveled on foot wading the rivers and creeks, was thin and feeble in very poor health, he stated that about a thousand men were seeking his life, from whom he had just escaped, does no regular work, will sometimes take a [mattor?] and dig for a day or two among the mountains, says he is looking for copper, never violent nor noisy, says very little unless spoken to, no suicidal tendency, admitted March 26 1858, address Wm. R. Utter, Ivy Log, Union Co., Ga.

633   **Wm. M. Warwick**, pauper patient from Lumpkin County, received May 1$^{st}$ 1857, eloped [blank], has been lurking among the mines most of the time since, is exceedingly cunning, has been brought within 30 miles of Milledgeville twice and escaped from his attendant, has twice escaped from the asylum, admitted March 31$^{st}$ 1858, see page 87.

634   **Wm. J. Rodgers**, pauper epileptic from Ware County, age 23 years, single, duration of epilepsy since childhood, is sometimes violent but usually easy to control, general health bad, admitted April 1$^{st}$ 1858.

635   **James M. Davis**, pay patient, formerly from Morgan County, now from Newton County, second admission to the asylum, was received Feb 15$^{th}$ 1857, see page 84, was discharged cured, remained well until February, since which time he has been growing worse, has been for some time in Barnesville on the assembling of one of the congregations for public worship in Barnesville, on last Sabbath he was found in the pulpit and refused to come out until it was promised he should preach to the negroes in the afternoon, which he did, he converses mostly on religious subjects, he is exceedingly noisy and restless, but not violent as yet, admitted April 5$^{th}$ 1858, address Joseph Reagan, Oak Hill, Newton Co., Ga., died Decr 10$^{th}$ 65.

636   **Mrs. Catherine Glassgoe**, pauper lunatic from Chatham County, age [blank] years, widow, no children, duration of insanity two years, has been in the Savannah hospital or jail nine months, cause of insanity unknown, admitted April 8 1858, died 6$^{th}$ May 1870.

637   **Mrs. Martha Dodgeon**, pauper lunatic from Cherokee County, married, has five children, youngest two years of age, her own age about 35 years, duration of insanity probably three years, possibly longer, cause became insane during recovery from a severe attack of illness, has eaten nothing,

is extremely feeble, not violent, admitted April 8[th] 1858, address John B. Garrison, Canton, Cherokee Co., Ga., died Sept 1[st] 1858.

638 **Mrs. Kate Nichols**, pay patient from Baldwin County, age [blank] years, married, has no children, last one became insane at time of its birth, the disease is hereditary, her father having been for many years insane, and remains so, admitted April 21 1858, discharged cured June 8, 1859.

639 **Lieut. Dudley Davenport**, pay patient from Savannah, age 30 years, single, duration one year or more, supposed cause masturbation which has been persisted in for 12 or 15 years, no known manifestation of unsoundness of mind, was perceived until about a year ago, when he engaged himself very unnecessarily in a personal difficulty with a gentleman in Charleston, all the circumstances showed very clearly his mind was disordered, has never shown any disposition to suicide and rarely any disposition to injure others, neat and cleanly in his habits, not destructive, is however very irritable and excitable and when opposed may be considered dangerous, he has been under medical treatment for six months, general health seems tolerable, received April 24[th] 1858, address H. M. Davenport, Savannah, Ga., discharged cured Feb 1[st] 1859. ($350)

640 **Adam Ellis**, pauper patient from Warren County, lunatic and epileptic, never married, had epilepsy when a boy, the convulsions ceased within a year, and he remained exempt from them for about eight years when they recurred and have continued every since, occurring at uncertain periods and irregular intervals for about twenty years, cause unknown, though when a child was in feeble health, eat dirt and human excrement, had however abandoned such habits and appeared in fair general health at the time of the recurrence of the convulsions, several of his mother's family were paralytic and died in that condition, recd. April 30 1858, died July 13 1858.

641 **Mrs. Allatha M. Lane**, pauper patient from Oglethorpe County, age 46 years, duration of insanity three or four years, cause unknown, health has been bad for a long time, has seven children, was very much troubled about the time she became insane on account of two sons who left home quite young, also lost a child about the same time, youngest child eight or nine years of age, strong suicidal tendency, shot herself with a pistol several years ago, ball entered the forehead, was supposed to have broken the skull but did not enter, usually quiet, has not been confined for long time, health not good, admitted May 4 1858.

642 **James H. Todd**, pauper epileptic from Walker County, age 27 years, duration of epilepsy fifteen years, mind was but little injured until about three years ago, sometimes violent noisy and dangerous, admitted May 4 1858, died June 28/60.

643 **Capt. Edwin Chambers**, pauper lunatic from Pike County, married, age 63 years, duration of insanity two years or more, cause pecuniary

embarrassment and apoplexy, is usually quiet but recently had two paroxysms of violent excitement, in the last of which he attempted to kill his wife with a carving knife, has been a farmer and shoemaker until two years past, has four children, all married except one, recd. May 5[th] 1858, died Nov 19 1859.

644 **Mrs. Elizabeth Holder**, of Cass County, was received Feb 3d, see page 111, but was found to be in a state of pregnancy and on that account sent home, her child was born fifteen days ago, her mind is no better, worse if any thing, than when she was carried home, a few days ago she succeeded in leaving her home unperceived, taking her babe a few days old with her and walked several miles through wheat fields, when she stopped she [wet?] to her waist, it did not seem to injure her in any way, recd. May 6 1858, August 11[th] discharged cured.

645 **Mrs. Lavinia Whitehea**, pauper lunatic from Baldwin County, was a patient in the institution some years ago (Mrs. Green), recovered and was employed for several years as an attendant, married, removed to the upcountry, remained there several years, returned here with her husband last winter seeking employment, was employed and a few weeks ago became again insane, admitted May 6 1858, discharged cured April 23 1859.

646 **William Baird**, pauper patient from Walton County, age about 55 years, widower, cause intemperance and loss of wife, duration 3 years, general health good, indifferent to personal cleanliness, destructive, will sometimes refuse food for several days altogether, admitted May 14 1858, died Sept 3 1858.

647 **Miss Elizabeth Bently**, pauper lunatic from Wilkes County, history unknown, admitted May 19 1858, died of marasmus 11[th] Nov 1873, notified.

648 **Mrs. Myley A. Delk**, pauper lunatic and epileptic from Liberty County, married, has been deserted by her husband, duration of epilepsy at least five years, has two children, youngest six years of age, admitted June 1[st] 1858.

649 **Chas. Brunning**, partial pay patient from Savannah, a German, his father was once a wealthy merchant in Breman but failed, he (Charles) came to Savannah, has been a clerk for Carr & Epping, a man of fine business habits and good character, supposed cause disappointment in love, a young lady to whom he was engaged and to whom he was much attached having deceived him, duration said to be less than three months, admitted June 5 1858.

650 **John Conner**, pay patient from Alabama, Tuskegee, expenses paid by the county, age 18 or 20 years, cause unknown, duration said to be a few weeks, occupation clerk, not violent or destructive but mischievous, admitted June 5 1858, address Batt. & Clark, Tuskegee Ala., discharged Oct 1[st] 1859. ($250)

651 **James Woodall**, pauper patient from Baldwin County, age 46 years, duration of insanity nine years, is said to have recovered and remained well several twice [*sic*] since the first attack, but most likely has never recovered from the first attack, is married, has [blank] children, is noisy and troublesome, but not violent, admitted June 8[th] 1858, discharged cured Sept 27 1858.

652 **Wm. Thomas Parks**, pauper epileptic from Cobb County, age about 24 years, duration at least ten years, admitted June 9 1858.

653 **Solomon Sweat**, pauper lunatic from Fulton County, age about 70 years, married, has several children, duration said to be nine months, supposed cause an injury received by being run over by a wagon, about ten months, admitted June 9 1858, died Sept 26 1858.

654 **Miss Patsy Warren**, pauper lunatic from Hall County, age 35 or 40 years, second admission, was an inmate of the asylum about six years ago, recovered and remained well until a short time since, cause unknown, is blind, has been almost totally blind for a year, admitted June 15 1858, address Joseph Read, Gainesville, Ga.

655 **Mrs. Mary Skinner**, pauper patient from Spalding County, age [blank] years, has five children, all grown, duration of insanity uncertain, probably some years, but very decidedly insane only a few months, suffers from the delusion that someone is seeking his [*sic*] life, admitted June 15 1858, address R. F. M. Mann, Griffin, died Oct 3/62.

656 **David Broderick**, pauper patient from Jones County, age about 45 years, duration of insanity about a year, cause paralytic attack which was the result probably of intemperance, occupation was once a stone cutter, for a year or two has been employed in the clerk's office of Jones County, is at this time in very bad condition, unable to walk or speak at all plainly, admitted June 19 1858, died August 24 1858.

657 **Jacob Keener**, pauper patient from Troup County, German, occupation cabinet workman, age [blank] years, duration of insanity [blank] years, cause unknown except it be an ardent desire to return to Germany with inability to do so, health at this time tolerably good, admitted June 19 1858, died 26[th] Nov 1878, heart disease, notified.

658 **Samuel L. Ward**, pauper patient from Fulton County, second admission, see page 5, was discharged Oct 1[st] 53, afterwards employed in the institution as miller, remained in its employ until last fall when his son induced him to go to Fulton County, had previously been addicted to habits of intemperance, the taste was revived and he fell, is now exceedingly noisy and wild, has been for several weeks confined in jail, admitted June 27 1858.

659 **A. B. Clark**, pay patient from Perry County, Alabama, age about 25 years, occupation has been going to school the most of his life, has been overseeing a little, duration of insanity about eighteen months, cause

onanism, the disease is hereditary, admitted June 25 1858, address Dr. Richard Clarke, Uniontown, Perry Co., Alabama, discharged cured April 1$^{st}$ 1859.

660 **Wm. W. Johnson**, pauper lunatic from Clinch County, age [blank], occupation farmer, was a patient in the asylum some years ago, entirely recovered, went home and remained well until a few weeks since, when he was found to be insane, supposed cause jealousy, is exceedingly noisy, violent, and destructive, admitted June 30 1858, address Millet Johnson, Magnolia, disch. cured Oct 1$^{st}$ 1858.

661 **Mrs. Jane Goodwin**, pauper lunatic from Pike County, age 50 or 60 years, married, deserted by her husband twenty years ago, has three children all grown, duration of insanity about twelve years, supposed cause about the critical period of her life her brother turned her out of doors, she seemed to be well prior to that, refuses food under the idea of poison, violent, very noisy and destructive, admitted June 30 1858, A. L. Hickman, Barnesville, Ga.

662 **Mrs. Harriet Ann Rusk**, of Nacodoches, Texas, wife of John C. Rusk, age 26 years, has four children, first indications of insanity within one month of the birth of her last child, which occurred on the 27$^{th}$ of November last, the first symptoms were an hysterical condition and the delusion that the cook was attempting to poison her, refusing to eat in consequence fro several days, she gradually grew worse but exhibited no tendency to violent excitement until eight or nine weeks ago, since which time she has been more or less excited every day, but uniformly rests well at night, never experienced previously any derangement of mind, some hereditary tendency suspected, she has been in feeble health for many years and more so now than formerly, has suffered for several years from prolapsus uteri and when not pregnant from dysmenorha and [*illeg. – menorrhagia?*], has been married nine years, has been treated by many physicians but with no apparent benefit, is the subject of very strong suicidal tendency, seeks most commonly to destroy herself by drowning or throwing herself from a window or from a height, is generally neat and cleanly in her habits, has shown no disposition to injure other persons, has generally a great unwillingness to eat, from the belief that it is not right she should eat, has had no menstrual or uterine disease since about three weeks after the birth of her child, when she had profuse and dangerous hemorrhage, received July 15 1858, if she dies her remains are to be sent to Mrs. McCall, or Dr. Collins at Macon, is to pay $600 per annum, died Sept. 1$^{st}$ 1858.

663 **Mrs. Martha Teat**, pay patient, second admission, was first received Sept 30$^{th}$ 1849, discharged cured Sept 2$^{nd}$ 1850, has since been in the asylum at Columbia, is very fleshy of a sanguine bilious temperament, admitted July 21$^{st}$ 1858, discharged cured July 11$^{th}$ 1859.

664 **Detif Hammeringham**, German, pauper patient from Muscogee County, occupation shoe maker, age [blank] years, duration of insanity [blank],

cause of insanity unknown, careless in his personal habits, not very filthy nor violent, admitted July 26 1858, died 23 Aug 1879, convulsions.

665 **Miss Patsy Noble**, pauper patient from [blank] county, age [blank], is blind, was an inmate in the asylum some years ago, has been insane for many years, admitted July 26 1858, died.

666 **Shadrack James**, pauper lunatic from Thomas County, single, occupation engineer, second admission, recovered and left the asylum in 1855, duration of second attack not known, but supposed to be recent, cause said to be disappointed love, admitted July 29 1858, died 9 Oct 1901, diarrhea.

667 **Mrs. Sarah Brady**, pauper patient from Baldwin County, married, has [blank] children, duration of insanity but a short time, admitted August 9 1858, discharged cured February 19, 1859.

668 **Patrick Moline**, partial pay patient from Bulloch County, age 25 years, single, native of Ireland, has lived in Georgia six years, duration of insanity four months, has a uncle insane, no immediate cause known, has shown no disposition to injure himself or others, is filthy in his habits, is quiet but does not sleep well, is disposed to wander off, will run away if he can, will not lie down, has been subjected to medical treatment but without benefit, has never drunk spirits, recd. August 11 1858, discharged cured Oct 1$^{st}$ 1858.

669 **Dr. Wm. W. Jones**, pay patient from Columbia County, age about 25 years, cause of insanity supposed to result from a [fatal?] difficulty with a schoolmate in Oxford College from close study and sedentary habits and disappointed expectations as to success in obtaining practice as a physician and subsequently the use of ardent spirits, duration of insanity about a year, has seemed rather eccentric all his life, is not disposed to suicide unless by poison, is disposed to be excited if crossed in any way, and would be likely to commit acts of violence but has threatened to do so only with a pistol, is very restive during the day and early part of the night, is sometimes disposed to destroy his clothes but nothing else, is disposed to be neat in his person and cleanly in his habits, has only been subjected to personal restraint for a few days and then confined to his room and his handstead, has been medicated only once, was then bled moderately, is naturally very chilly in cold weather, has used tobacco excessively, received August 14, 1858, Mr. F. A. Jones, Wrightsville, Ga., died 9 May 1893, cancer, notified.

670 **Miss Caroline Maclin**, partial pay patient from Prattsburg, about 41 years of age, single, cause of insanity supposed disordered health, has for some years been dyspeptic, and for many years has been the subject of mennorhagia, the discharge often so profuse as to enfeeble her very much, duration of disease the symptoms of derangement of mind were not such as to attract attention until last November, but probably existed some time previously, has not attempted suicide but has frequently

threatened during her paroxysms of excitement to destroy herself by taking laudanum, is not destructive and is very cleanly, most prominent delusions relative to the necessity of saving money and the fear she will come to want, received August 17, 1858, discharged cured Dec 28, 1858.

671 **Mercy Morgan**, pauper idiot and epileptic from Clinch County, age [blank] years, admitted August 17, 1858, died Nov 16 1858.

672 **Jackson Hargroves**, pauper idiot and epileptic from Bibb County, duration from childhood, admitted August 24 1858.

673 **John L. King**, pauper lunatic from Floyd County, widower, disease hereditary, immediate cause probably intemperance, duration but a short time, is violent and noisy, received Sept 2$^{nd}$, discharged cured Oct 1$^{st}$ 1858.

674 **Mrs. Tabitha Tidwell**, pauper lunatic from Paulding County, age about 90 years, widow, duration of insanity unknown, cause unknown, admitted Sept 3$^{rd}$ 1858, died Sep 1858.

675 **Madison Flanders** patient from the penitentiary, idiot, a convict from Worth County, term of imprisonment May 2$^{nd}$ 1860 [or 1868], admitted Oct 18 1858.

676 **Andrew McMickin**, lunatic from the penitentiary, convict from Cass County, term of imprisonment was to expire Sept 1859, admitted Oct 18 1858, discharged May 10 1859.

677 **Thos. H. Burch**, pay patient from Russell County, Alabama, age about 37 years, married, has 3 children, duration of insanity not exceeding a year, cause irregular life and pecuniary embarrassment, health tolerably good except nervous headaches at uncertain intervals, no hereditary tendency known to exist, his insanity is exhibited in acts of mere childishness, has shown no disposition to commit any act of violence, is believed to have had a convulsion of some sort last week, is filthy and destructive, received Oct 29 1858, removed by his friends June 11, 1859.

678 **Wm. Terry**, pauper patient from Fulton County, age about 60 years, but little is known of history, has been an inmate of the asylum at Columbia, S.C., duration of insanity unknown, but certainly several years, thinks he is commissioned by heaven for some great reformation, is neat and cleanly in his habits, not destructive, received Nov 4 1858, died.

679 **Miss Sarah Bishop**, pauper idiot from Campbell County, age [blank] years, received Nov 5 1858.

680 **Enoch Murphey**, pauper lunatic from Forsyth County, age 26 years, married, has 3 children, has been separated from wife 8 years, duration according to his statement since 1847, was committed some years ago but was not brought to the asylum, cause unknown, occupation teacher of vocal music, some of his friends were afraid of him but has never been known to commit any act of violence, was confined in jail some years ago,

and again recently for several weeks at each time, admitted Nov 6 1858, address [blank].

681 **Mrs. Martha Chance**, pay patient from Montgomery County, age [blank] years, was an inmate of this institution some years ago, improved while here and was taken home by her friends, her name was then McRae, she afterwards married in a few months, her husband committed a [perjure?] (forgery or counterfeiting) for which he was sentenced to the penitentiary, this cause a relapse, admitted Nov 10 1858.

682 **Green Walker,** partial pay patient from Washington County, idiot and epileptic, age 33 years, had epilepsy from early infancy until seven years of age, had no from that time until he was twenty years of age, at which time they recurred and have not ceased to occur at uncertain intervals since, is very fleshy and is in the enjoyment of good general health, received Nov 11, 1858, died Feb 11 1859.

683 **Augustus C. Whitworth**, pauper idiot from Madison County, age about [blank] years, received Nov 14, 1858.

684 **Elizabeth Whitworth**, pauper idiot from Madison County, sister of the above, age about ]blank] years, received Nov 14 1858, Sept 23/60 died.

685 **Mrs. Susanah Cooper**, of Macon County, Alabama, age about 32 years, married, has five children, youngest six months of age, duration of insanity on this occasion about 3 months, after the birth of her first child was three or four months insane, that child died two days after birth, has at sometimes destroyed her clothing, has never attempted suicide but has spoken of it, does not attempt acts of violence except toward her husband when he would not allow her to do as she wished, has been a professor of religion twelve years or more, is a member of the Baptist church, her most prominent delusions are that spirits of God has left her forever and that her husband and baby are dead and she does not recognize any of her family, there is supposed to exist some hereditary tendency to insanity, she has been under treatment but with no manifest benefit, she has rarely been induced to take medicine, received Nov 15 1858, address G. W. Cooper, Guearyton, Macon Co., Ala., died Jan 31$^{st}$ 1859, had recovered of insanity but died of fever.

686 **John Hare**, pauper patient from Webster County, age about 30 years, single, duration uncertain but supposed to have existed to some extent at intervals for three years, cause believed to be intemperate habits, native of Ireland, has lived in southwest Georgia about 4 years, his employment has always been ditching, health generally good, had intermittent fever last fall, has been confined in jail occasionally and in Sumter County was whipped, has no suicidal tendencies, has attempted to strike and kick persons, is not destructive, is careless but not filthy, received Nov 17, 1858, eloped January 27$^{th}$ 1867, returned August 1$^{st}$ 1867.

687 **Mrs. Louiser A. Selman**, pay patient from Floyd County, widow, age 47 years, has eight children, youngest six years old, was insane two years

ago, was not as bad as now, became better, was regarded as well until last July, is violent, has attempted suicide, some symptoms of insanity shown at the time of her husband's death 4 years ago, cause ill health, has had a cough for several years, has suffered from uterine disease, became insane at the critical period of life, admitted Nov 17, 1858, address James Selman, Ducktown (Dirttown), Ga., if she should die send her remains to Rome, Ga., died of consumption and mania Feb 21$^{st}$ 1859.

688   **Miss Susan Holman**, pay patient from Randolph County, age about 20 years, duration of insanity about two months, supposed cause religious excitement, she has been a professor of religion five or six years, a member of the Baptist church, no hereditary predisposition known to exist, her health has been generally good, no suicidal tendency, not destructive, always neat and cleanly, has labored under mennorhagia and dysmennorhagia, received Nov 22 1858, address David Holman, Cuthbert, Ga., discharged cured April 21 1859. ($250)

689   **Miss Nancy Ford**, pauper patient from Cass County, single, age about 40 years, cause unknown, duration of insanity unknown, received Nov 23 1858.

690   **Wm. Pope**, pauper lunatic from Bibb County, age 38 years, duration one month, supposed cause ill health, he is at sometimes much excited and injures himself by throwing himself against the floor and wall, has threatened suicide if he could get a knife, he is disposed to be neat and cleanly but sometimes destroys his clothing, his health has been poor for a long time, has suffered from stricture for ten years, has been operated upon several times, is readily controlled by mild judicious efforts, had an attack of fever last all, received Dec 4$^{th}$ 1858, Mr. Pope has practiced onanism for year and is believed to be impotent, disch. Dec 23$^{rd}$ 1858.

691   **Thomas W. Howell**, pauper patient from Randolph County, married, has two children, duration of insanity about a year, supposed cause a fall from a horse which rendered him senseless for some hours, causing hemorrhage from his ears, soon after this he lost an important debt, nearly his all, is a member of the Baptist church, threatened to ill his wife that he might marry another woman, admitted Dec [blank] 1858, address Mrs. Mourning M. Howell, Georgetown.

692   **John Lawrence Carson**, pay patient from Greene County, age about 20, single, duration a short time, received Dec 9 1858, address Mrs. C. F. Carson, Greensboro, Ga., discharged cured Feb 4 1859.

693   **Carnaby Veal**, pauper epileptic from Paulding County, age [blank] years, duration unknown, admitted Oct [blank] 1858, address F. Carter Moore, Dallas, Ga., died Apl 13/61.

694   **Mrs. Louisa Grant**, pauper patient from Houston County, age [blank] years, duration of insanity [blank], cause unknown, received Oct [blank] 1858, Mrs. Gt was found wandering through the country, she says her name is Mrs. Grant, daughter of Mr. Stephens, died June 16/60 [or 61?]

695    **Mrs. Lidia Langham**, pauper lunatic from Pike County, age 46 years, has been married and separated from her husband 18 or 20 years, has 3 children all grown, duration of insanity believed to be only ten days, was badly burned about the face when 9 years old, was insane about 18 years ago about 3 or 4 months but remained rational from that time until ten days ago, has lived with her son in law, has been employed weaving, washing, &c., for some time previous to the attack suffered from an offensive discharge from her ears and was very deaf, since the attack her hearing has become very acute, she has been in a constant state of excitement during the entire time, has slept scarcely at all and has not eaten during time what would amount to an ordinary meal, is very filthy and destructive, has had some medical treatment but without benefit, is supposed to be in a state of constipation now, received Dec 13 1858, died quite suddenly Dec 24 1858.

696    **Edward J. Bacon**, pauper epileptic from Stewart County, age about 35 years, married, has children, duration of epilepsy 3 years, the attack occurs about every two weeks, received Dec 21 1858.

697    **Robert C. Gray**, of Gadsden County, Florida, lunatic, age about 30 years, single, is a native of Twiggs County, but has resided in Florida for eighteen years, occupation farmer, duration of insanity not certainly known, is believed to have been gradually becoming so for several years, has for two years been roaming about the country, cause masturbation, he is usually orderly and quit though sometimes excited, has never shown any disposition to commit acts of violence, not destructive, is rather filthy in his habits, his mother was insane for years, admitted Dec 22$^{nd}$ 1858, died Oct 14$^{th}$ 1861.

698    **David Eubanks**, of Gadsden County, Florida, lunatic, age about 27 years, native of South Carolina, has lived for 18 or 20 years in Florida, single, duration of insanity believed to be 8 years or more, was kept chained for a year, a small hut was then built for him of very heavy split logs without doors or windows, leaving a small opening through which his food and water were passed, and a small opening in the floor at one corner, in that place and under such circumstances he has spent the last 4 years without clothing or bedding as everything of the kind given him was immediately torn up, the sheriff states that when he went for him the stench of the place was intolerable, cause masturbation, is yet very violent, destructive, and filthy, and persists in the practice supposed to be the cause of his insanity, received Dec 22$^{nd}$ 1858, died Augt 25/59.

699    **John P. Henry**, pay patient from Chattooga County, age about 51 or 52 years, married, his wife and several children [*illeg.*], earliest indications of derangement of mind observed about 3 years ago, continued however to attend to his business correctly and was not considered insane until about six months ago, cause primarily very decided hereditary predisposition, immediate exciting cause loss of property and embarrassment in his business, he is quiet and readily controlled, not at all filthy in his habits, does not rest well but has a good appetite, not disposed to commit acts of

violence, is believed to have some tendency to suicide, at one time went to the river, it was thought for the purpose of drowning himself, at another secreted a rope and denied having seen it, received Dec 25 1858, address John W. Powell, Newnan, Ga., discharged cured March 25 1859.

700 **Mrs. Anna Presswood**, pauper patient from Catoosa County, age about 35 years, is married but her husband deserted her about 4 months ago, has six children, all girls, duration of insanity uncertain, about three years ago contracted syphilis from her husband and suffered very much, lost an eye, is believed to have entirely recovered, received Dec 28 1858, address Hon. Spraybury, died 4 April 1878, dropsy, notified.

701 **Isaac W. Peeler**, pauper lunatic from DeKalb County, age about 25 years, duration of insanity two years or more, cause unknown, was a young man of intelligence and fair education, has never been intemperate, was born in Jasper County but brought up in DeKalb, for some years prior to the occurrence of insanity was employed in working on a farm and teaching school, has for a long time used tobacco excessively, was absent from March to December of last year, travelling in the southwestern states, has never been married, is not noisy or disposed to commit acts of violence, has no suicidal tendency, has for months been peculiarly taciturn, would rarely speak when spoken to and for a week past has not been heard to utter a word, general health good, had however a protracted attack of intermittent ever last spring, no hereditary predisposition believed to exist, received Jan 2$^{nd}$ 1859, address E. T. Chapman, Lithonia, Ga.

702 **Frederick Bryan**, of Barber County, Alabama, age about 25 or 26 years, married, has four children, has been insane about 18 months, cause believed to be overheat in cutting wheat and drinking freely of cold water before becoming cool, is quiet and orderly, never disposed to acts of violence, no suicidal tendency, is very cleanly in his habits, rests well, general health seems good, complains that his head often aches, came to the asylum willingly, paid his board &c. himself, received Jan 6 1859, discharged cured May 24$^{th}$ 1859.

703 **Martha Ella Oglesby**, from Elbert County, pauper epileptic, age 10 years, duration over 2 years, is paralytic on her left side and partially on the right, admitted Jan 6 1859, address Shale Oglesby, died 4$^{th}$ April 1869, marasmus. ($12.00).

704 **Elizabeth L. Adams**, from Jasper County, partial pay patient under certificate of Inferior Court, age about 29 years, single, been insane for 14 years, supposed cause a severe and protracted attack of illness, was in the early stage of insanity very violent and was confined for about a year since she requires only to be looked after by a servant, is now in a state of dementia, is always quiet, is often filthy, never destructive, is sometimes indisposed to eat but can be persuaded to eat ~~but can be induced~~, does not get up at night but often does not sleep well, general health feeble, has had an aunt and brother insane, the brother was once an inmate of this institution, received Jan 6 1859, dead.

705 **Peter Finelle**, pauper patient from Muscogee County, says he is from South Carolina, age unknown, duration [blank], cause [blank], received 8 Jany 1859.

706 **Mrs. Harriett Edwards**, pauper patient from Oglethorpe County, deaf, dumb, and insane, age about 30 years, married to a mute, has had four children, two have died, youngest living 18 months old, has been insane for three or four years, immediate cause unknown, very strong hereditary predisposition, her father and several other members of her family have been insane, is cleanly but destructive and disposed to throw everything into the fire, does not rest well at night, her general health is apparently good, her husband and herself were both educated at Hartford school for mutes, and he was at one time an assistant in the school at Cave Spring Georgia, received Jany 17 1859, address Henry P. Shackelford No. 6, S. Broad St., Atlanta, Ga., died 7 Nov 1887, chronic diarrhea, notified.

707 **James Sewell**, pay patient from Coweta County, age about 50 years, married, farmer and mechanic, duration a year or more, cause believed to be intemperance, is usually quiet and has shown no disposition to commit acts of violence toward any one but his own family, is rather filthy in his habits, general health declining, received Jan 19 1859, if he dies his remains are to be sent in a burial case to Mrs. James Sewell, Newnan, Georgia, died April 1$^{st}$ 1859.

708 **Kenneth C. Greene**, pauper lunatic and epileptic from Terrell County, age about 35 years, has been married but his wife left him some years since, had no children, duration of epilepsy 12 or 14 years, cause unknown, is usually quiet and orderly, sometimes otherwise on the occurrence of the convulsions, not filthy in his habits, convulsions usually occur at night, received Feb 2$^{nd}$ 1859, died 8$^{th}$ July 1876, notified Ordinary.

709 **Miss Selina Pinsen**, pauper lunatic from Floyd County, age about 27 years, single but has a child six or seven years old, duration of insanity 12 years, cause unknown, is usually quiet and not filthy, general health rather feeble, other members of the family are believed to have been insane, received Febry 3$^{rd}$ 1859.

710 **Morris Brewer**, pauper lunatic from Cass County, age about 22 years, has been imbecile to some extent from birth but has grown worse for some years back, has occasional paroxysms of excitement in which if annoyed he will strike one, not disposed to wear his clothes, not destructive but filthy, had his leg badly burned lying out at a log heap some two months ago, not often noisy, is restless at night, received Feb 7 1859, died May 14 1859 of dysentery.

711 **John Keaton**, partial pay patient from Carroll County, age about 45 years, single, duration of insanity about 18 years, cause unknown, hereditary predisposition traceable, had a sister insane who died in this institution, does not speak, has not for 8 years, organs of speech not diseased, rather filthy, received Feb 9 1859.

712 **Mrs. Mary E. Walker**, pay patient from Uniontown, Perry County, Alabama, age about 39 years, married, has 4 children, youngest 10 years old, duration of insanity about 6 years, cause unknown, hereditary predisposition very strong, her grandfather and several other members of her family have died insane, has suffered from scrofula for many years, her general health very poor, received February 11, 1859, removed July 10[th] 1862.

713 **Mrs. Mary C. McMahen**, pauper patient from Lee County age between 55 and 60 years, has had 11 children, 10 are living youngest 15 years old, duration of insanity 10 or 12 years, cause unknown, was all her life the subject of very violent sick headache, occurring very frequently until since the birth of last child, about 3 years after that event the attacks became less frequent and evidences of disorder min became manifest and as the interval between the attacks became more prolonged her mind became worse, now she rarely ever has headache but the condition of her mind is worse than ever before, has a brother insane, is usually quiet and orderly, neat in her habits and not disposed to commit acts of violence, received February 11 1859.

714 **Mrs. Frances M. Edwards**, pauper patient from Gordon County, second admission, was received here Oct 6[th] 1856 and discharged Sept 16 1857, see page 76, relapsed in a few weeks, as been much worse for four months, has had one child since her discharge from the institution which is now about 5 months old and is her eighth child received February 14[th] 1859, address M. B. Edwards, Calhoun, Ga.

715 **Mrs. Elizabeth Logan**, pauper lunatic from Spalding County, age about 55 years, widow, has been twice married, had three children, lost all of them, first noticeable symptoms of insanity soon after the death of her first husband 6 or 7 years ago, having previously lost her children, her last husband was a very old man, died 3 years ago, was no doubt insane when she married him, has been worse for three years and been growing still worse recently, has been at times chained to prevent her running about the country, cause supposed to be loss of husband and children, address Wilson S. Burnes, Griffin, Ga., admitted March 9 1859.

716 **Hugh Rusk**, lunatic from Jackson County, Florida, age about 45 years, has been twice married, now a widower, his last wife and 3 children died within two years past, duration of insanity quite uncertain, but his friends have not considered him insane for more than four months, had mania [potir?] last March, cause primarily doubtless very intemperate habits for twenty years, the immediately exciting cause loss of cotton and tobacco on the river, and temporary embarrassment, his general health has been usually good, except chronic dysentery from which he suffered occasionally until the last three months, he is usually quiet, has threatened violence but never committed any such act ecept the whipping of a negro severely without any reason, he is very neat and cleanly in his habits, usually rests well in the latter part of the night, never has been confined in

any manner, received March 4 1859, address Dr. Wm. Yarbrough, Marianna, Florida, died Decr 22$^{nd}$ 1864.

717 **Peter Lee**, pauper lunatic from Chatham County, age about 45 years, married, has a wife and two children, occupation laborer, duration of insanity about 18 months, cause supposed to be the loss of a child, very quiet and orderly, has no disposition to commit acts of violence, attempted suicide twice by seeking to drown himself, general health usually tolerably good, received March 13$^{th}$ 1859.

718 **Mrs. Mahala Barns**, pay patient from Dallas County, Alabama, lunatic, age 50 to 55 years, married, has three children, all grown, duration of insanity more than twenty years, cause unknown, has been an inmate of the asylum at Lexington Ky for fourteen years, general health appears good, is usually tolerably good, is usually tolerably quiet, is not destructive or filthy, received March 26 1859, address Merrit Barnes, Selma Ala.

719 **Daniel H. McCollum**, pauper lunatic from Cherokee County, age 25 years, single, occupation farmer, duration of insanity about 7 years, cause supposed effects of a very serious attack of typhoid fever, has been generally quiet and orderly until within the last six months, since which time he has been quite ill natured, has threatened violence toward his mother and sisters, raised a lightwood knot to kill his mother, has never shown any disposition to commit acts of violence toward any one else, is cleanly in his habits and not destructive, received March 30 1859, communicate with Mr. Williams, bookkeeper at the penitentiary, died Jany 5$^{th}$ 1862, advised Mr. Williams.

720 **H. G. Curtis**, pay patient, lunatic from Lower Peach Tree, Wilcox County, Alabama, age about 23 years, single, has been engaged for some years in the study of medicine, duration of insanity probably two years or more, cause believed to be masturbation and dyspepsia, has been excitable from the commencement but much worse in that respect for the last six months, and so constantly disposed to commit acts of violence, as to render it necessary to confine him in a log hut built for the purpose, he is not disposed to tear clothing or bedding but will break up articles of furniture, has not recently exhibited any suicidal tendency, when first attacked he did, is habitually [*illeg.*], sometimes particularly in damp weather noisy at night, received April 1$^{st}$ 1859, address Dr. C. C. Curtis, Lower Peach Tree, Ala., died [blank], has been subjected to very little medical treatment.

721 **Mrs. Jane Waller**, pauper lunatic from Laurens County, age about 28 years, married, was abandoned by her husband last winter, has three children, the youngest a mulatto about 4 years old, duration of insanity something over two years, cause domestic difficulty and severe illness, in which there were prominent symptoms of cerebral disease, is usually quiet and orderly, is not noisy or filthy, general health has appeared good since the attack about referred to, received April 6$^{th}$ 1859, address Francis Thomas, Esq., Dublin, Ga.

722   **Miss Mary C. Ebbs**, pauper lunatic from Cass County, age about 18 years, was the subject of derangement of mind four years ago which was believed to have resulted from the death of her mother, was then insane for four or five months without change, after that she grew better and became capable of attending to the ordinary duties of the household and remained in such a state until within the last two weeks when she became suddenly much worse and has continued so, she has never appeared entirely well since first attacked four years ago, is now very violent and noisy, has decided suicidal tendencies, has endeavored to cut her throat and also to hang herself, is often disposed to assault other persons, is very destructive and filthy, cause of the recent change for the worse in her condition supposed to be the influence of her father marrying a second wife and moving to Arkansas, received April 12 1859, address Dr. N. T. Bridges, Pine Log, Cass Co., Ga., discharged.

723   **John Brumbilo**, pauper idiot from Pike County, age 28 years, has had epilepsy since childhood but did not have a convulsion during the last two winters, but had them during the summer, received April 19 1859.

724   **Mrs. Rhoda R. Parker**, pay patient lunatic from Jacksonville, Florida, married, age about 53 years, has three children all grown, duration of insanity supposed to be about three weeks, cause not known unless dissatisfaction in relation to her removal this spring from Vermont to Florida, her family are all very nervous and excitable people but no example of derangement of mind known to exist except in the case of one of her daughters who has been twice an inmate of the McLean Asylum but is now entirely well, general health of Mrs. Parker very feeble, her nervous system is very much disordered, received April 20 1859, address E. F. Parker Esq., Jacksonville, Florida.

725   **Allen Mabry**, pauper lunatic from Lincoln County, age about 70 years, married but has separated from his family at least twelve years they being in Alabama, during which time he has lived alone on his brother's plantation doing his own cooking, &c., was arrested last fall for assault, having attacked a man with a stick but was not put upon his trial, has not attempted violence toward himself but has occasionally toward other people, duration of insanity probably many years, received April 30 1859, died July 29 1861.

726   **Mrs. Martha Ann Brown**, partial pay patient from Macon County, age about 22 years, duration of insanity about nine months, cause influence of parturition [childbirth] and loss of her infant within the first week after the birth of her child the lochia were arrested and no discharge has taken place from the uterus since, was in the care of physicians for three months, was bled, cupped, and purged freely but without any benefit, when first attacked she threatened suicide and sought to drown herself but manifested no disposition to effect it in any other way, is not disposed to offer violence to others, is not destructive or filthy, early in the attack burned some articles of her clothing but has not for several months exhibited any tendency to do mischief, general health rather feeble, has

recently had intermittent fever, last paroxysm occurred on Sunday last, received May 4[th] 1859, address James M. Brown, Oglethorpe, Macon Co., Ga.

727   **John Donaldson**, pauper lunatic from Lumpkin County, age about 58 years, has several children, all grown but one who is about four years old, has been insane for six or seven years, cause the cessation of free discharge from hemorrhoids to which he had been accustomed for years, general derangement of health and paralysis, has no suicidal tendencies but is often disposed to commit acts of violence toward others, has attempted to kill his wife, is generally however quiet and orderly, is neat and cleanly in his habits and not destructive, does not sleep well, received May 5 1859, address Dr. N. T. Howard, Dalhonega, Ga.

728   **Joel Smith**, pauper lunatic from Pearce County, age about 29 years, married, has been insane three months or thereabouts, cause disordered health and religious excitement, joined the Baptist church about twelve months ago and since then has been greatly concerned and excited about the state of some of his relatives who are very wicked, is very constantly violent and noisy and is generally disposed to attack any one who may be near him, had pneumonia about a year since and has never entirely recovered from the effects of it, since he became insane has suffered several times from haemoptysis, does not rest well, received May 5[th] 1859, address Benj. Minchew, Blackshear, Pearce Co., Ga., discharged cured June 16 1859.

729   **Daniel Gillis**, partial pay patient from Montgomery County, age about 32 years, single, occupation farmer, duration of insanity about six years, cause supposed to be injuries received by a blow from a stick of timber, he was assisting to raise the timber when it fell, striking him on the back and knocking him over, he falling with his breast across a cart tongue, was probably insane from the time the injury was received but about two weeks afterwards was palpably insane so that he had to be confined for a day or two, when he became exceedingly weak and probably suffered from partial paralysis, was thought at one time to be dying but gradually recovered strength and motion, since that time his mind has been disordered but he becomes worse, usually about once a month, at first the paroxisms lasted only a few days, but for several months they have lasted as much as two weeks, has been at times violent, having tried to shoot one brother and attempted to cut another with a knife, not suicidal, not destructive, admitted May 10 1859, address Merdock Gillis, Little York, Montgomery Co., Ga., is certified to be worth $140 dollars, discharged cured.

730   **Matthew Stephens**, pauper lunatic from Lumpkin County, age about 62 years, married, no children, cause injury to head by a fall from a horse, duration four years, after the injury was senseless for two weeks, and since that time his mind has been deranged, is very violent, often excited and dangerous, filthy but not destructive, received May 11 1859, address Mrs. Sarah Stephens, Dahlonega, Ga.

731   **Mrs. Bathsheba Lynum**, Wilcox County, Alabama, age about 44 years, married to second husband, has had one child some ten years ago which was stillborn, was very low after the birth of the child, has had a tumor on her back for twenty years, was treated by a "cancer doctor," [*quotes in record*] the tumor is said to be nearly healed, was insane in 1851, duration of first attack five months, seemed to be cured by removal from her then place of residence, her husband having had a difficulty with his employer, went to a strange community (he being an overseer), she seemed to be well in a week after the removal, cause supposed by her friends to be religious excitement and anxiety for the salvation of her husband, and jealousy, she of her husband, he and she are both members of the Baptist church, she says, and with good reason, the cause of her present condition was the suicide in a fit of delirium caused by drunkenness of the son of her husband's employer, she and the mother of the young man having been exceedingly anxious about his salvation and desirous for him to be a preacher, duration about two months, has been treated, was depleted by cups and cathartics without benefit and then stimulants were tried with like result, is often excited and sometimes violent, received May 14 1859, address Dr. Wm. M. Clarke, Rehoboth, Wilcox Co., Ala., her husband's name is James L. Lynum, discharged cured August 2$^{nd}$ 1859.

732   **Thos. Cummings**, pauper lunatic from Richmond County, age about 35 years, single, duration of insanity some eight years, supposed to have resulted from sun stroke, is usually quiet an orderly but occasionally becomes excited and is then disposed to assault anyone about him, is not filthy in his habits but very indifferent about cleanliness, no suicidal tendency, general health is good, rests well at night, is never noisy, received May 16$^{th}$ 1859, address [blank], died 8 Apr 1894, Jaundice.

733   **Thomas Blackburn**, pauper lunatic from Floyd County, age 46 years, single, occupation groom, duration of insanity unknown, cause unknown, general health rather feeble, received May 17, 1859, address [blank], discharged and went home with his wife June 18$^{th}$ 1867.

734   **Miss Susan W. Sims**, pay patient from Macon, age about 18 years, condition congenital, has learned to read and write to some extent, her sisters menstruated at eleven years of age, she did not until sixteen years of age and has been irregular ever since, the discharge occurring at intervals of two or three months or longer, had three epileptic convulsions in a period of six months three years back but nothing of the kind has occurred since, seems to have difficulty in voiding her urine but never suffers from excessive retention, she has threatened suicide, received May 25$^{th}$ 1859, address ~~Erastus Kirtland, Macon~~, Mrs. W. H. Bray, Eufaula, Ala., died 24 June 1911, apoplexy, buried here.

735   **Miss Catherine S. Moore**, pauper lunatic from Wilkes County, age about 32 years, single, duration of insanity four years, cause death of friends and menstrual suppression which existed for some months about the commencement of her attack, but she has been regular as to the periods ever since, her general health usually feeble and the subject always of

habitual constipation, usually rests well but often otherwise, eats very irregularly, often has passed five days without eating and again eats inordinately, has now eaten nothing for two days and drank no water since leaving home until she reached the asylum, is always excited in company or where she can see or hear anyone, is very destructive occasionally, has threatened suicide but never attempted it, is disposed to commit acts of violence to others only when efforts are made to force her to do anything she does not wish, she is not filthy in her habits but very careless on such subjects, received June 1$^{st}$ 1859, address Mrs. S. L. Bolton, Maxey, Geo.

736    **Miss Emeline E. Pearson**, formerly Mrs. E. E. Tullis, lunatic from Pike County, Alabama, recently removed from the asylum at Nashville, age about 46 years, has never had any child, duration of insanity ten or twelve years, cause hereditary predisposition developed by religious excitement, has three or four brothers who have been or are insane, was born in North Carolina and remove to Alabama in 1851 and was married in July of that year to Mr. Tullis who in about four or five months discovered that she was insane and that she was insane before her marriage, file a bill S.C.&C., her general health unusually good, often very much excited, not destructive, sometimes disposed to commit acts of violence, captious and exacting, was in the asylum at Nashville about 18 months, removed unimproved, received June 2$^{nd}$ 1859, address D. A. M. Perota, Pike Co., Ala.

737    **Thos. Lasseter**, pauper lunatic from Clayton County, single, age about 47 years, duration of insanity 18 years, cause supposed to be an attack of typhoid fever, occupation farmer, not violent, destructive, filthy, noisy, or suicidal, labors under general paralysis and has done so for three years past, his bowels are often disordered, received June 4$^{th}$ 1859, address James Homes Jr., Jonesboro, Clayton Co., Ga.

738    **Miss Mahulda Coward**, pauper lunatic from Pickens County, second admission, was received in June 1857 and discharged in October of the same year cured, remained well [blank], cause of relapse [blank], for former history see page 89, received June 5$^{th}$ 1859, address Mr. Allredd.

739    **Mr. Thomas J. Ingram**, pauper lunatic from Carroll County, age [blank] years, second admission, was removed by his friends, for former history see page 80, received June 15, 1859, eloped 8$^{th}$ Dec 1867.

740    **Mr. Robt. Lee**, lunatic from Jefferson County, age 27 years, single, his mind has been feeble all his life, but unequivocal manifestations of insanity accompanied with a disposition to commit acts of violence never observed until last fall, cause hereditary influence, is usually quiet and orderly, is sometimes excited and disposed to assault persons about him, not filthy but careless on such subjects, is rarely ever noisy, received June 16 1859, address Mrs. Amy Lee, Pope Hill, Jefferson Co., Ga., to pay $14 per an.

741   **Mrs. E. M. Dyer**, pauper lunatic from Catoosa County, age 27 years, married, has never had a child, has been married seven years, it is believed by her family that her husband gave her medicine for the purpose of preventing conception, duration two years, she is now in a state of dementia and of partial paralysis, seems unconscious of everything around, does not attend to the calls of nature, is usually constipated, has not urinated for thirty seven years, supposed cause ill treatment received from her husband, no hereditary tendency known, received June 20 1859, address [blank], died July 25[th] 1860.

742   **Mr. Harvey W. Nancy**, lunatic from Columbus, merchant, age about 45 years, married, duration of insanity six to eight months, cause believed spinal [*illeg.*] and diminution of accustomed hemorrhoidal discharge, earliest indication of disordered health a constant tendency to sleep whenever he sat down, within the last ten days has become liable to paroxysm of violent excitement, particularly when opposed in anything, has been always very temperate, for some five months past has taken under prescription of a physician two drinks of brandy or whiskey every day, is not generally noisy or filthy, does not usually sleep well at night, received June 21[st] 1859, address Mrs. Elizabeth Nance, Mr. M. M. Nancy or L. G. Bowers, Esq., guard.

743   **Mrs. Jane Allen**, lunatic from Pike County, widow, age about 64 years, was brought to this institution on 2[nd] of August 1854, the subject of most violent mania, the history then furnished of her case was to the following effect, vis., "Age about sixty years, became insane twenty years back or more, has never been regarded as altogether sound since, but not in such circumstances as to render it necessary to restrain her, until some two years back, cause unknown, general health feeble," on that occasion she remained in the institution nine months, and was sent home entirely restored, has remained at home in a sound state of mind until about seven months back when evidences of returning insanity were observed, her general health has been good through out the period since she went home and she has acquired flesh to a considerable extent, but she has walked very little, has recently complained much of pain in her back, her mind is now very greatly disordered, she is very excitable and destructive and filthy, sometimes noisy and often disposed to commit acts of violence upon any person about her, has not recently been allowed to have a knife or other article with which she could do mischief, received July 7[th] 1859, address A. S. Allen, Griffin, Ga., if she should die her remains must be sent in a metallic burial case to A. S. Allen or Edward Foster, Griffin, Ga.

744   **Mr. Joseph Edwards**, pauper lunatic of Richmond County, age 58 years, married, has been a farmer, worked in a tan yard and for a few years past has been a root doctor, has at some times drank regularly but never regarded as intemperate, cause of insanity unknown, no suicidal tendency, not disposed to offer violence toward others except when he is opposed, not filthy but careless, received July 12[th] 1859, address Clerk of Inferior Court, Augusta, Ga.

745 **Mr. Arthur McGrath**, (pronounced McGraw), pauper lunatic and epileptic of Richmond County, age 22 years, railroad laborer, has had epilepsy for three years, when a child of five or six years a wheel of a carriage passed across his forehead, and when about 12 years old experienced a sunstroke, has convulsions very frequently, when the paroxysms are very violent he becomes sometimes greatly exited and it is very difficult to restrain him, they usually occur during the day, is quiet and orderly and readily controlled except when the paroxysms occur, and is only at such times at all dispose to be destructive or filthy, received July 12 1859, address Clerk of Inferior Court, Augusta, Ga.

746 **[no name] Mitchell**, pauper lunatic from Liberty County, nothing known of him, was found wandering about on an island in the county subsisting upon whortle berries, says he is one hundred eighty years old, speaks very unintelligibly, received July 13$^{th}$ 1859, died 20$^{th}$ Feby 1869, marasmus.

747 **John W. McDaniel**, lunatic from Walker County, age about 29 years, occupation farmer, single, duration of insanity two years, cause supposed to be disappointed affection, is not known to have been intemperate, has been under irregular treatment, six months back was dispose to offer violence to others when opposed but has not recently shown any such disposition, is not specially filthy but very careless in relation to such matters, never noisy but does not usually rest well, general health always good, received July 13 1859, address Jno. McDaniel, his father and guardian, Lafayette, Walker Co., Ga., to pay $250 per annum, sixty of which is received, died 20 Nov 1891, notified.

748 **Miss E. C. Dorman**, lunatic and epileptic from Fayette County, single, about nineteen years of age, epilepsy first occurred about seven years ago, cause unknown, did not menstruate until she was sixteen years old and has been irregular ever since, has not now menstruated for twelve months, frequently complains of heat and pain about her head, convulsions occur regularly, has threatened suicide when excited and endeavored to get a knife, under such circumstances is sometimes disposed to offer violence to others, is occasionally very noisy, usually sits at the table with her family, is not generally filthy, but is careless and indifferent on such subjects, and when she has convulsions often has involuntary olvine discharges, does not rest well, received July 21$^{st}$ 1859, address Richard Dorman, Fayetteville, Ga., died 18$^{th}$ Sept 1870.

749 **Eldridge S. Cash**, lunatic from DeKalb County, age about 45 years, single, duration of insanity more than ten years, cause hereditary influence, quiet orderly and cleanly, was an inmate of this institution from May 30$^{th}$ to December 1th 1850, was then taken away by his friends, somewhat improved but by no means well, received July 23$^{rd}$ 1859, address Washington Cash, Decatur, Ga.

750 **Benj. Donald**, lunatic from DeKalb County, age 25 to 30 years, no information in relation to his case, was found some six weeks back in an unoccupied house three or four miles from Decatur in a state of the

utmost destitution and manifestly insane, has been since confined in the Decatur jail, has made no attempt to commit suicide but has frequently wished he was dead, has been uniformly quiet, says he came last from Alabama and came from Sumter District So. Ca. three years back, received July 23rd 1859, address Alexander Johnson, Clerk of the Inferior Court, Decatur, Ga., eloped Apl 13/62, returned May 6/62, died 19th Nov 1868.

751 **Mrs. Cornelia Teel**, lunatic from Harris County, age about 38 years, married, has several children, youngest about six years old, duration of insanity about three years, cause supposed bad conduct of her husband, she had an uncle who was insane but recovered after the lapse of a year, is usually quiet and orderly, occasionally otherwise but has only once committed any act of violence, she then struck a negro woman who was pulling her out of the kitchen, has never been at all destructive or filthy, has smoke excessively, received July 2y6 1859, address Erasmus Teel, her husband, or Calvin Teel, her father, Hamilton, Harris Co., Ga.

752 **Mrs. J. A. Dixon**, from Quitman County, pauper, age about 45, married, has seven children, youngest about 5 years old, duration of insanity 20 years, but for most of the time has been able to attend to ordinary household duties, about 12 years ago had a severe attack at which time she attempted suicide, got better of that attack and remained better until about two months ago, about which time her minister reproved her for wearing hoops to church, citing her to a passage of scripture to prove the sinfulness, it gave her a great deal of trouble, she seemed to think of nothing else for some time and soon showed symptoms of mania, original cause supposed to be jealousy, probable hereditary tendency, her sister died insane, has attempted to injure her family but no else, has not attempted to injure herself except by throwing herself on the floor, is not filthy or destructive but will sometimes take off her clothing, is lecherous and sometimes obscene, received August 4th 1859, discharged Novr 27th 1860.

753 **Mrs. Anna Parker**, from Wilkinson County, widow, no children, age 59 years, duration of insanity 12 or 15 years, has been blind of one eye for several years, became entirely blind in the other only a few weeks back, usually quiet and orderly, general health feeble, received July 21st 1859, address [blank], died Sept 10/60.

754 **Jefferson Brand**, lunatic and epileptic from Taylor County, age 22 years, single, duration of epilepsy six or seven years, cause unknown, an interval of two years occurred between the first and second convulsion, became then frequent twice a week or more frequently, has been under medical treatment, general health previous to first convulsion very good and for two years or more continued so, since then has been declining, no hereditary predisposition known but has a cousin who is insane, is not filthy or destructive but is frequently disposed to commit acts of violence, tried to shoot his brother, received August 12th 1859, address Thos. D. Brand, Butler, Ga., died Augt. 4th 1861.

755 **Henry Redding**, from Emanuel County, pauper epileptic age about 27 years, has been in the county two years, says he left a wife and child in Florida, duration seven years or more, has been worse for two years, is sometimes violent and dangerous, is destructive but not filthy, admitted August 27th 1859, discharged July 24th 1860.

756 **Mrs. Mary D. Perkins**, lunatic from Burke County, married, has three children, youngest twelve months old in June last, duration of insanity seven or eight months, cause succeeded a long protracted attack of typhoid fever, in which she was for some weeks in a comatose state, is not violent, destructive or noisy, has no suicidal tendency, is neat and cleanly, no hereditary predisposition believed to exist, her health up to 55 was extraordinarily good, since rather feeble, decidedly more so since the attack of fever, was born in Burke County, has not menstruated since the birth of her last child, before her last pregnancy was believed to be laboring under disease of the womb, received Spet 7th 1859, address N. M. Perkins, Millen, Burke Co., Ga., or Mr. W. M. Reynolds (Guardian), Lawtenville, Burke Co., Ga., 1887 Jany 17, remains to be sent home, telegraph Mrs. W. M. Reynolds, Millen, Ga.

757 **Lewis Daniel**, pauper lunatic from Randolph County, age about 40 years, was once married but his wife ran off with another man some fifteen years ago, duration of insanity eighteen years, gradually becoming worse, disease believed to be hereditary, general health feeble, has lived for ten years past in a hut he put up himself about ten feet square where he has voluntarily remained except when driven out by hunger, has lately shown a disposition to do mischief with fire, is not noisy or destructive , not very filthy but very careless, received Sept 14th 1859, address Wm. Johnston, Cuthbert, Ga.

758 **Mrs. Daisy Strickland**, widow from Appling County, lunatic, age about 50 years, duration of insanity about 4 years or perhaps more, cause believed to be the neglect and ill treatment of her husband who died four years back, general health not good, is sometimes excited but never disposed to commit any act of violence, never raves but is noisy occasionally by loud singing, easily controlled, never destructive or filthy, is rather specially disposed to habits of neatness and cleanliness, received Sept. 14th 1859, address Mr. Elijah Ogdam, Holmesville, Appling Co., Geo., died of paralysis April 25th 1860.

759 **Miss Julia Gunn**, of Houston County, age 22 years, single, duration between 3 and 4 weeks, cause supposed to be watching and anxiety in attending upon a sick aunt, excessive use of snuff, quinine, &c., is represented to have spent days and nights constant novel reading and extravagant use of snuff, is believed to be suffering from some menstrual irregularity, general health uniformly good until five or six weeks, since which time she has had more or less feverishness, is disposed to constipation, suffers much from pain in the back of her head and heat of head, sleeps well every other night, on the intermediate night is restless and noisy, is very loquacious but does not rave, is neat and cleanly in her

habits, when she is excited will break up things, is not otherwise destructive, is not disposed to do herself injury but has threatened violence to others and should be carefully watched when she has a knife or scissors, is laboring under the delusion that everything is dirty, received October 10th 1859, discharged cured Feb 21st 1860.

760 **Sylvanus Stokes**, pauper lunatic from White County, age 31 years, single, duration of insanity five years or more, cause believed to be spiritual rappings, &c., came from Tennessee to White County six months ago, was an inmate of the asylum at Dayton, Ohio, for eighteen months, is said to have escaped from there, is a man of some education, is rather filthy in his habits, has no disposition to injure himself, not disposed to commit acts of violence, is likely if has opportunity to do mischief with fire, burned a house in White County by direction of spirits, general health usually good, always quiet, never raves, received Oct 12th 1859, address Clerk Inferior Court, White County, Ga., Mt. Jonah, note, is sometimes disposed to attack persons around, which attacks are usually very sudden.

761 **Mrs. Eliza J. C. Little**, pay patient of Harris County, age 42 years, married, has nine children, youngest about six years old, duration of insanity about eight years, suppose cause disordered health of many years duration, has made excessive use of tobacco smoking and [*illeg.*] with snuff, has been subjected to medical treatment and traveled quite extensively without benefit, is usually quiet, but occasionally paroxysms of excitement in which she is profane and obscene, has no suicidal tendency, no disposition to offer violence to anyone, not destructive or filthy, general health tolerably good, menstruates regularly and seems worse at that time, received Oct 14th 1859, address Rev. J. J. Little, Whitesville, Harris County, Ga., discharged March 29th 1860.

762 **Mrs. Sophia M. Jones**, pauper patient Thomas County, age 35 years, has been married, her husband has been divorced from her, has one child ten years of age, at the birth of child placenta was not delivered, had convulsions and was insane for some time probably has been ever since, but was thought to have gotten well, her husband was divorced on the ground of her doing nothing for him and her being of bad disposition, received Oct 31st 1859, address Hugh [McCa??], Boston, Ga., died Mar 29th 1861.

763 **John B. Saltmarsh**, Catawba, Alabama, age about 31 years, single, cause of insanity injury of head and masturbation, duration about 15 years, some decided hereditary predisposition exists, is usually quiet and orderly, but is sometimes destructive and excited, careless in reference to cleanliness, is not disposed to do violence to himself or others, Nov 8th 1859, address [blank.

764 **Green B. McCrary**, pauper patient from Warren County, age about 30 years, occupation laborer, has taught school, single, duration of insanity four months, is not known to be violent but has made one attack on mother and brother, was put in jail under a peace warrant in September, is

very taciturn, admitted Nov 8[th] 1859, address Wm. J. MCrary, Tannville, Warren Co., Ga..

765   **Wm. E. Lazenby**, part pay patient from Warren County, single, age 27 years, occupation school teacher, was insane in 1854, was confined at home for several months, cause of that attack supposed to be masturbation, duration of present attack some months, was teaching three months ago, cause of present attack probably masturbation, has threatened suicide by hanging, exhibits fear of persons around him, is cleanly, not destructive but careless, admitted Nov 8[th] 1859, address Robert H. Lazenby, Thompson, Ga., Feb 16[th] 1860, Mr. L. seems about well, denies very solemnly that masturbation was the cause of his attacks, attributes the last attack to care of a large school with sedentary habits.

766   **Wilbur E. Collier**, pay patient from Clarke County, Alabama, age 19, single, has been eccentric all his life, but manifested mind, no indication of decided aberration of intellect until last May, first indication was a refusal to give up money which his mother had given him to keep for her, and afterwards presenting a gun heavily loaded at his brother, suffered with severe pain in his head last fall, was probably insane to some extend last spring, was a year, very indifferent to personal neatness and cleanliness, is laughing to himself for several days and is again angry and cross for a like period, has been confined only for a few days, admitted Nov 25h 1859, address A. M. Collier, Suggsville, Ala., died of inflammation of bowels, May 8[th] 1860.

767   **James R. Hendry**, of Gadsden County, Florida, age 25 or 38 years, single, occupation farmer, duration of insanity three years last April, cause unknown, was intemperate and had been for some years, but was not regarded seriously so, has shown a disposition to commit acts of violence, but has not actually done so except in case of a man who chained him &c., is quiet and cleanly, has never been treated for insanity, general health usually good, received Nov 2[nd] 1859, address James M. Smith, Quincy, Florida, died of diarrhea Sept 15[th] 1862.

768   **Walter S. Withers**, from Fulton County, age about 22 years, single, occupation moulder in a foundry, duration of insanity twelve months or more, cause intemperance and hereditary predisposition, but no decided manifestation until four or five weeks past, when not drinking is quiet and orderly and decent and cleanly in his habits, received Dec 4[th] 1859.

769   **Francis W. Warner** (under certificate), lunatic and epileptic from Bibb County, age about 18 years, has had epilepsy since he was eighteen months old, convulsions occur at uncertain periods, longest interval he has experienced is four weeks, always quiet and orderly and cleanly, received Dec 10[th] 1859, died Nov 6[th] 1862.

770   **Thomas W. King**, from Franklin County, age about 30 years, pauper, duration of insanity uncertain, probably for years, health feeble, received Nov 20[th] 1859.

771 **Miss Elizabeth Holder**, pauper epileptic from Walton County, age 25 years, has had epilepsy since childhood, has convulsions every week or two, is often violent and dangerous, is in a low state of health, is in a state of dementia or most likely idiocy, received Dec 11[th] 1859, address Gideon Welborn, Monroe, Walton Co., Ga., died 7[th] Feby 1874, notified.

772 **Mrs. Nancy A. Filigim**, pauper patient from Greene County, married, has had seven children, youngest eighteen months old, age 36 years, duration of insanity six years, has had two children since she has been insane, during pregnancy with the first she seemed to have entirely recovered, and was better During her last pregnancy, but each time became worse soon after delivery, is worse about the menstrual period, first attack was probably caused by disordered menstruation, has threatened to cut her throat abut has never attempted violence to herself or others, not destructive or filthy, received Dec 11[th] 1859, address J. W. Filligim, Greensborough, Ga.

773 **Miss Louisanna Lee**, from Jefferson County, received under certificate to pay $15.00 per annum, age 25 years, she is one of five children, all of whom except one are feeble minded, has a brother in this institution, her father was insane, the oldest child has more mind than the others, her mind has become decidedly worse during the past year, is disposed to wander off, but is not violent but sometimes noisy, received Dec 13[th] 1859, address J. T. Mullen, Louisville, Ga.

774 **Mrs. Patsey Fields**, lunatic from Hall County, widow, with three children, age about 35 years, duration of insanity some eight years, but has gradually grown worse, her nephew, Henry Faulkner, was restored from such a state in this institution, she has threatened to drown herself but never attempted it, is frequently excited at night, noisy and destructive but not filthy, received Decr. 19[th] 1859, address Benj. Faulkner, Polksville, Hall Co., Ga., discharged Oct 1[st], left on Nov 8[th] 1861.

775 **James D. Barker**, pay patient from Coosa County, Alabama, has been a school teacher, clerk, and farmer, married, has three children, youngest child three years old, is a member of the Methodist church, cause of insanity onanism, has been the victim of the habit since he was ten or eleven years of age, first symptoms of insanity noticed in 1851, about which time he married by the advice of his brother, seemed better for some time but soon relapsed and has been getting gradually worse for a long time, has threatened suicide and carried laudanum for the purpose, has threatened to lie down before the cars on the railroad, received Dec 21[st] 1859, address Dr. W. H. Baker, Bradford, Coosa Co., Ala., discharged Nov 20/60.

776 **John S. McDonald**, pauper patient from Columbia County, single, age about 35 years, duration unknown, had always been feeble minded, is sometimes violent, cause onanism, received Dec 28[th] 1859.

777 **Mr. A. K. Leonard**, pay patient from Talbot County [no information].

778 **Mrs. L. E. Cole**, pauper patient from m, widow, has several children, youngest four years of age, age about 36 years, history not known, except that some years ago her husband was killed, his murderer was afterwards hung, has probably been insane for years, is noisy and violent, admitted Dec 30th 1859, died 24th April 1875, marasmus.

779 **James H. Wheelus**, pauper lunatic and epileptic from Upson County, age 15, duration unknown, received Dec 31st 1859, address Henry Wheelus, Culloden, Ga., died Augt 27th 1861.

780 **Howell E. Chitty**, lunatic and epileptic from Henry County, Alabama, history of the case to be furnished by Dr. W. J. Johnson, received Dec 31st 1859, discharged 7th Sept 1868.

781 **Ivin U. Black**, pauper lunatic from Union County, age about 30 years, occupation farmer, cause of insanity unknown, duration unknown, is always quiet and orderly, never has attempted violence, does not sleep well, is of [costine?] habit, no hereditary predisposition, none of the family specially intelligent, received Jan 9th 1860, died of dysentery July 8th 1862.

782 **Verginia O. Wolfe**, pauper epileptic from Effingham County, age about 14 years, has been subject to convulsions since she was about 4 years of age, first brought on by a fall from a cart, has an uncle in the institution, received Jan 10th 1860, address C. L. Wolfe, Eden, Effingham County, Ga., died Augt. 20th 1860.

783 **Sarah K. Himeby**, pauper idiot from Effingham County, age about 18 years, has had epilepsy, which was probably the cause of loss of mind, is an orphan, received Jan 10th 1860, address Richard E. Himeby, Springfield, Ga., removed 17th July 1877, improved.

784 **Anderson R. Bishop**, pauper epileptic from Campbell County, age 12 years, duration of epilepsy six years, has a sister in the asylum who is also the subject of epilepsy, received Jan 13th 1860, address Reuben Bishop, Fairburn, Campbell County, Ga.

785 **Mrs. Mary Wood**, pauper lunatic from Coweta County, married, has had two children, youngest is five months old, has been married between three and four years, an aunt on maternal side is insane and has been for many years, first symptoms noticed two years ago last August, seemed hysterical and suffered with nightmares for some time but soon suffered from illusions and delusions, thought persons around her intended to take her life, this occurred seven months after the death of her first child, and ten months after its birth, since which time she had never menstruated, finally became pregnant and was better until after the birth of the child, since which time she has gotten much worse, seems now to have lost all affection for her babe, not violent or suicidal, but often excited, received Jan 17th 1860, address James N. Wood, Lodi, Coweta [County], Ga.

786 **Miss Sarah Garman**, lunatic from Macon, age about 26 years, single, duration 3 years or more, cause unknown, more [*unclear*] history will be

furnished by Dr. Searcey, received Jany 21$^{st}$ 1860, address Mrs. M. H. Garman, Macon, Ga.

787  **Mrs. H. S. Lewis**, lunatic from Augusta, age 41 years, married, has three children living, youngest child she has had, if living, would now be eight years old, duration of insanity some two months, thought not decidedly manifest until ten days back, four months back had a stroke of paralysis afflicting principally her tongue, suffers from general nervous disturbances, general health quite feeble, probably the subject of the constitutional disturbance incident to the critical period, &c., she is usually quiet but sometimes impatient, shown no tendency to suicide, is not destructive but disposed to strip herself, is cleanly, received Jany 23$^{rd}$ 1860, address Wm. E. Sikes or F. W. Reagan, Augusta, died Nov 28/61.

788  **Nathan Chambers**, pauper lunatic from Clayton County, age about 25 years, occupation farmer, duration of insanity 8 years, cause supposed to over heat from cutting wheat or from an attack of sickness resulting therefrom, was kept at home and was not confined for years, but has become very violent since about Christmas, seems now to be laboring under violent mania, was addicted to intemperance to some extent before his first attack, asks for spirits now, destructive and violent, no suicidal tendency, has a cousin insane, received Jan 25$^{th}$ 1860, died of maniacal exhaustion, May 22$^{nd}$ 1860.

789  **William Moss**, lunatic from Henry County, third admission, age 57 years, occupation laborer, has five children living, one died an inmate of the asylum some years since, four are now admitted with him, two as lunatics and two as idiots, has a son in Henry County who is said to be insane, Mr. Moss is now suffering from violent mania, a few days since tore down his smoke house, burnt his meat, ditched his year and planted cotton seed in the woods, was brought to the asylum in chains and handcuffs, is very violent and rather filthy, received Jan 27$^{th}$ 1860, discharged.

790  **Almida Moss**, from Henry County, daughter of William Moss, pauper lunatic, age 18 or 20 years, duration of insanity three years, rather violent and noisy, received Jan 27$^{th}$ 1860, died Aug 28$^{th}$ 1861.

791  **Betsy Ann Moss** (sister to Almida), pauper lunatic from Henry County, age about 16 years, duration of insanity unknown, condition very similar to that of her sister, received Jan 27$^{th}$ 1860, discharged.

792  **Martha Moss**, pauper idiot from Henry County, age 30 years, is quite small, received Jan 27$^{th}$ 1860, discharged.

793  **Josiah Moss**, pauper idiot from Henry County, age about 20 or 22 years, received Jan 27$^{th}$ 1860, died Nov 23 1861.

794  **Jasper R. Henry**, pay patient from Calhoun County, Alabama, age 31 years, married, has two children, duration of insanity nearly three years, cause unknown, for the first six months seemed but little affected, read the Bible constantly and was very melancholy, since then has had a flow

of spirits, is easily excited and sometimes threatens violence but has never committed any, has threatened to fire the premises of different persons, has an aunt, Mrs. Holt, who has been insane, she recovered at this institution, Mrs. H. is a sister of his mother, received Feb 4th 1860, address Wm. Henry, Weehoga, Calhoun Co., Ala., discharged Nov 23rd 1861.

795  **Mr. F. Midlam**, lunatic from Augusta, married, has several children, cause close application to business without recreation or rest, has been for many years general agent for Georgia Rail Road, hereditary tendency, his mother died insane, received [blank].

796  **James W. Skinner**, pauper epileptic and lunatic from Spalding County, age about 25 years, single, duration of epilepsy from childhood, hereditary predisposition, usually quiet day & night, convulsions occur at least once a week without any special regularity as to day or night, is cleanly, never violent, received Feb 6th 1860, address Robert Skinner, Griffin, Ga.

797  **Mrs. Ann White**, pauper lunatic and epileptic from Floyd County, age about 20 or 30 years, duration of epilepsy since childhood, very little is known of her case, she has been in Floyd County about two weeks, received Feb 8th 1860.

798  **Jefferson Eubanks**, lunatic from Gadsden County, Florida, age about 28 years, single, occupation farmer, no indication of insanity known until six months ago, cause unknown, hereditary predisposition known to exist, is usually quiet and orderly, has not attempted violence toward himself or others, cleanly and decent, does not sleep well, received Feb 10th 1860.

799  **Miss Julia Ann Sanders**, lunatic from Gadsden County, Florida, age 19 years, single, duration 14 years, cause inflammation of the [brain? – *unclear*], she is usually quiet and orderly, has never been confined, received Feb 10th 1860, address James M. Smith, Sheriff.

800  **Sarah Ann Harrall**, pauper epileptic from Twiggs County, age 22 years, single, duration of epilepsy 8 years, had paralysis when about 3 years of age, has never recovered from it, suffered from scrofulous disease, about 9 years ago several pieces of bone were taken from her arm and shoulder, as the abscesses were healing spasms came on, which gradually growing worse have become now severe convulsions is sometimes irritable but not violent, received March 9th 1860, discharged.

801  **Susan Drew**, idiot from Talbot County, age 31 years, received March 20th 1860, discharged.

802  **Martha Drew**, idiot from Talbot County, sister of Susan, age 20 years, received March 20 1860.

803  **Mark R. Lewis**, lunatic from Clark County, Alabama, age about 36 years, single, duration of insanity about 20 months, occurred suddenly, cause unknown, occupation farmer, was always steady moral and temperate and for several years past a member of the M. E. Church, no hereditary

predisposition, health always rather feeble, when about 12 years old was knocked senseless by the fall of a [*unclear*] of a tree, seemed however to recover from it in a few days, received March 20$^{th}$ 1860, address Wm. B. Lewis, Choctaw Corner, Clarke Co., Ala., died 15 Oct 1889, dropsy, notified.

804 **W. A. Woodburn**, pay patient from Florida, was removed from the institution in February, condition unchanged, returned March 21 1860.

805 **James L. Hinton**, pay patient from Meriwether County, removed from the asylum by his friends but his family became afraid of him and have returned to the asylum, received March 28$^{th}$ 1860.

806 **Elizabeth J. Whitehead**, pauper lunatic and epileptic, age about 35 years, single, duration of epilepsy, since childhood, paroxysms occur every week or more frequently, cause unknown is usually quiet and orderly and decent in her habits, received March 30 1860, address John G. Pollock, care of Duval Adam, Perry, removed unimproved 15$^{th}$ July 1879, returned 7$^{th}$ Aug 1879, died February 1899, epilepsy.

807 **Mrs. Sarah Cramer**, pauper lunatic from Walker County, was formerly a patient, has experienced a return of mental only four weeks ago, cause disordered health, received April 2$^{nd}$ 1860, address James W. Creamer, Lafayette.

808 **James Slaughter**, idiot from Harris, age about 10 years, received April 11$^{th}$ 1860.

809 **Mrs. Mary Murphy**, pauper lunatic from Fulton County, widow, about 45 to 50 years of age, duration of insanity, cause unknown, received April 28$^{th}$ 1860.

810 **Andrew J. Pledger**, pauper lunatic from Clayton County, single, laborer, age about 27 years, duration of insanity eight or ten years, probable cause masturbation, some hereditary taint, has a cousin Mr. Chambers now in the asylum, very careless in his personal habits, not violent, but his family have been unable to control him, received May 5$^{th}$ 1860, address Josiah Chambers, Jonesboro, Clayton Co., Ga., eloped June 7$^{th}$ 1862, died 21 May 1920, bronch. pneumonia, burial here.

811 ~~**Jules Lefler, alias [Bernadotle?]**, pauper patient from Dalton, native of Germany, age about 40 or 45, single, occupation book keeper, has resided in the county seven or eight years, has at times shown evidences of insanity ever since he has been in the country, but at other times appears perfectly rational, unless some offense was given has never attempted violence, his health has been generally good but during paroxysms of derangement becomes very thing, does not eat bacon, is not fond of meat, is cleanly and orderly in his habits, is disposed sometimes to burn his clothing, when a paroxysm is coming he becomes unsocial and will not shake hands with any one, received May 10$^{th}$ 180, address Lewis Bender,~~

~~Dalton, Ga.~~, died 1 June 1887, note, the above scratching out said to have been done by the patient himself.

812 **John M. Wade,** of Warren County, age 25 or 30 years, married, has one child, farmer, duration of insanity unknown but supposed to be recent, was for several years a school teacher but has not taught for about six years, has a cousin who died insane, within two years has become a regular drinker and has occasionally been intoxicated, has also taken to use tobacco, had never used either before, is not generally disposed to commit acts of violence, made threats against his wife, has threatened suicide, is cleanly and not destructive, received May 10 1860, address [blank], discharged Augt 20th 1860.

813 **Elizabeth J. McMillin**, idiot and epileptic from Lumpkin County, received May 14th 1860, address McMillin, Dahlonega, Ga., died Jany 10/61.

814 **John S. Davis**, epileptic from Fannin County, age 42 years, married, has seven children, duration of epilepsy three or four years, has been much worse for two years, convulsions occur two or three times a month at which times he sometimes has seven or eight, cause supposed to be intemperance, is frequently violent, has to be confined with a belt and chain, received May 15th 1860, address Wm. H. Davis, Pierceville, Fannin Co., Ga., removed Jany 15th 1863.

815 **Joseph Smith**, pauper lunatic from Chatham County, age about 25 years, has been in Savannah jail for six or eight months, history unknown, was taken up as a vagrant and found to be insane, received May 16, 1860, died 20 Jany 1891.

816 **Telitha Woodall**, pauper lunatic from DeKalb County, married, duration of insanity five or six years, became insane about the critical period of life, age 52 or 53 years, sometimes violent and noisy, not filthy but careless, received May 22nd 1860, address Hamilton G. Woodall, Decatur, Ga., died 29th Oct 1867.

817 **Mrs. Elizabeth Kitchen**, pauper lunatic from Thomas County, has one child who is grown, age about sixty years, duration of insanity probably twenty five years, cause became insane during child bed, the child was removed by instruments, is now talkative and lively but her condition varies, she is sometimes in her present condition for a year or two and passes from that to a melancholy frame of mind during which she has very little to say, in her present condition when excited uses very bad language, but is ordinarily decent in her habits, has attempted suicide by hanging and has frequently threatened violence to those around her, her father died insane, died of starvation, other relatives have probably been insane, received May 19th 1860, address J. W. Walker, Thomasville, Ga.

818 **Mrs. Eliza A. Bigham**, pauper lunatic from Fulton County, age 27 years, married, has two children, youngest six weeks old, duration of insanity five weeks, cause puerperal, her last labor seemed perfectly natural and she continued well for a week except that there was no secretion of milk,

on that day 8[th] day she seemed hysterical, told her husband "she had been delirious and that she had told him she was cold when in fact she was very warm, and that the remedies used had been of great disadvantage," nothing had been given her and she had made no complaint, in a few hours she was raving and her mind has not been clear since, is sometimes violent and obscene, for several weeks seemed to sleep none, but for a week past has slept tolerably well every other night, no suicidal tendency, no hereditary predisposition, before labor her extremities were very much swollen and have not entirely subsided yet, received May 25[th] 1860, address William Bigham, Macon, Ga., discharged.

819 **Thos. R. Williams**, pauper lunatic from Forsyth County, age about 38 years, duration of insanity three years, married but separated from his wife, has been in California for about six years, was a merchant before going to California, cause of insanity unknown, was temperate before going to California, has been otherwise since, is usually quiet and orderly, is noisy at night, has not shown any disposition to commit acts of violence, is not filthy, received May 28[th] 1860, address his brother John L. Williams, Cumming, Forsyth Co., Ga.

820 **Mrs. Kate Nichols**, pay patient from Baldwin County, second admission, see page 119, was discharged cured June 8[th] 1859, remained well until about three weeks ago, she relapsed quite suddenly, gave birth to a daughter near three months since, labor was natural and convalescence rapid without an unpleasant symptom, health has been apparently excellent, cause of relapse unascertained, received June 1[st] 1860, discharged Jany 1[st] 1861, returned and discharged 10[th] Dec 1867.

821 **Mrs. Elizabeth Roberts**, pauper lunatic from Jackson County, married, age about 50 years, youngest child 15 years old, duration of insanity about 4 years, cause unknown, usually quiet and orderly, sometimes excited and noisy, has made threats to burn houses, is ordinarily cleanly in her habits, received June 3[rd] 1860, died 6[th] Aug 1871, consumption, not informed, not knowing who to write to.

822 **Dr. Thos. S. Park**, pay patient from Harris County, discharged Augt 13[th] 1860.

823 **Mr. Morrim**, pay patient from Savannah, died Sept. 6[th] 1861.

824 **Mr. Scott Blakey**, pauper lunatic from Spalding County, age 24 years, single, farmer, cause of insanity inflammation of the brain, duration about 7 or 8 months, manifested by singular conduct, has threatened suicide upon no particular plan, and has made no attempt, has threatened violence toward his father and mother, suffered much from headache for weeks, finally fever supervened, had a severe attack with symptoms of inflammation of the brain, upon his recovery from that attack became free from headache but as he recovered his mind became worse, is restless at night, does not eat anything but cornbread and water, received June 6[th] 1860, died Septr. 14[th] 1860.

825    **Mr. Wade H. Lester**, lunatic from Cobb County, age about 30 years, married, occupation planter, cause of insanity exposure to the sun, on the first day of June was seining for four hours bareheaded, ten years ago from excessive labor as a clerk and loss of sleep, he got into a state of unnatural excitement with some indications of mental derangement, shortly afterwards experience an attack of fever, recovering from that he was found to be mentally sound, the entire period being six to eight weeks, in the present attack he is the subject of acute mania, has been treated by physicians in Atlanta as they say <u>heroically</u>, among other remedies was bled very freely, has been usually in a state of almost constant excitement and has slept very little and eaten very little, is violent and destructive, received June 10<sup>th</sup> 1860, address Robt. B. Lester, Americus, or by telegraph Jno. R. Hill, Esq., Macon, died June 16<sup>th</sup> 1860.

826    **Mr. Doctor F. Long**, pauper lunatic from Rabun County, age about 25 or 30 years, single, cause epilepsy, duration of epilepsy ten or twelve years, supposed to have resulted from an injury received when a boy by the rolling over him, is usually quiet and orderly, has threatened acts of violence but has committed none, decent, quiet, cleanly, has convulsions at uncertain intervals, received June 11<sup>th</sup> 1860, address Mrs. Mary Long.

827    **Mrs. Ann Armstrong**, pauper lunatic from Washington County, age 28 years, married, has had five children, four are living, duration of insanity about 2 years, was brought to the hospital last fall, was then pregnant and for that reason was not received, has since given birth to a child Jan 1<sup>st</sup>, has been quite feeble since, the child lived two months, cause of insanity unknown, was in feeble health at the time of the attack, complained of headache and tremulousness, was in the habit of using tobacco to excess, occasionally violent, does not sleep well, received June 11<sup>th</sup> 1860, address A. C. Armstrong, Worthens Store.

828    **Wilson M. Chapman**, pauper lunatic from Whitfield County, age about 22 years, single, occupation harness maker, duration of insanity 15 months, cause supposed to be religious excitement and study, he is usually quiet and orderly, is tolerably cleanly in his habits, disposed to constipation, received June 14<sup>th</sup> 1860, address Edwin E. Chapman, Dalton, Ga.

829    **Bertrand Zachary**, lunatic from Fulton County, age about 38 years, married, dealer in furs, duration of insanity about 6 years, was in California mining when a stone fell upon his head, which stunned him causing insensibility for twelve hours, he returned to Georgia and those intimately acquainted with him could discover that there was some change in the condition of his mind, he remained in much the same state until four weeks back when he became suddenly worse, about that time he was made sick by getting very wet, and suffered greatly with his head, he was also the subject of very considerable religious excitement, he has not required to be restrained until about 10 days back, had a fit last Friday morning and had some slight return, has attempted to commit acts of violence upon his wife and others, is usually quiet but talks loudly and preaches at night sometimes, sleeps only tolerably well, has eaten very

little recently, is not destructive, is decent an cleanly in his habits, has been treated but with no manifest advantage, received June 14[th] 1860, address Lewis Zachary, Covington, Ga., discharged Septr. 13[th] 1860.

830 **Bridget Tracy**, pauper lunatic from Muscogee County, received June 18[th] 1860, address James M. Huges, Columbus, Ga., died June 16[th] 1861.

831 **Alexander Green**, pay patient from Walker County, married, has a wife and two children, seven or eight years ago was attacked while at school during the spring of the year, was violent and had to be confined, during the next spring he recovered and has remained apparently well until last spring when he was again attacked, no cause is known, no hereditary taint, tubercular disease is hereditary, not violent, but has threatened violence, his mind is in a low state, received June 25 1860, address Jesse Green, or Dr. G. M. Kerns, Ringold Ga., discharged Jany 15[th] 1862.

832 **Miss Elizabeth Ansley**, lunatic from Warren County, native of Georgia, age 32 years, duration of insanity 15 years or more, cause gross abuse of her uncle by beating her severely with a cowskin &c., having given her as much as 250 lashes at one time, generally health unusually good, menstrual function ordinarily health, sometimes too protracted then she is worse, usually quiet and orderly, no suicidal tendency, not disposed to commit acts of violence, cleanly, does not use obscene or profane language, received July 10[th] 1860, died 14 July 1897, marasmus.

833 **James Armour**, pauper lunatic from Bibb County, age about 30 years, married, occupation engineer on Central Rail Road, was insane for some weeks four years back, was then subjected to no treatment except confinement in jail, duration of this attack two weeks, suppose cause domestic disturbance, hereditary predisposition suspected, has been in jail for a week, has been violent and destructive but not filthy, not suicidal, cut a Negro with a knife and attempted violence upon others, received July 12[th] 1860, address Mrs. Jane Armour, Macon, Ga., eloped Oct 5[th] 1860.

834 **William Lewis**, lunatic from Cass County, native of England, age 36 years, single, occupation clerk, was formerly a patient in this institution, was restored, remained well for three years, when returning to intemperate habits he became again insane, his father being averse to sending him to the asylum he was subjected to treatment at home by physicians in the neighborhood who bled and purged him very liberally, has remained in the same state ever since, now about 9 years, is generally quiet and orderly, is sometimes excited and very profane, never disposed to commit acts of violence, not destructive or filthy or careless, received July 15[th] 1860, received Apl 1/61 partially restored, returned Apl 28/62 in much the same condition, Dr. Powell says 14[th] Feby 1890, his brother Mr. Nathaniel D. Lewis, Stilesboro, Ga.

835 **Miss Margaret K. Sherman**, pauper patient from Baldwin County, single, age 35 years, occupation school teacher, third attack, first attack

when about 22 years of age, remained insane 3 or 4 months, recovered entirely, second attack last July, lasted until about Christmas, began teaching in January in Wilkinson County, has taught in the college in Madison, and also at Penfield, taught last year in Atlanta, had a large school and took boarders, her father and mother afflicted, over exertion probably cause the attack, her health has been tolerably good, last attack was first observed about 3 weeks ago, this seems to be the first attack, had been closely confined with her school, at times violent, received July 21$^{st}$ 1860, discharged.

836   **Wm. Connelly**, McIntosh County, age about 45 years, married, has two children, one about 4 years old, about 2 years ago was found to be insane, was taken up by the Inferior Court and kept in jail for about a month, seemed to recover entirely, was set at liberty and remained well until about 4 months ago when he became worse, drank to excess for many years, was coroner of his county, had two troublesome cases of inquest which excited him very much, after each one of which took a spree which resulted in insanity, both attacks being produced by the same sort of circumstances, is suicidal, has attempted suicide twice, once with a razor and once with a pen knife, received July 25$^{th}$ 1860, address Wm. J. Donnelly, Darien, Ga., care of John Smith, City Marshal, discharged Sept. 27/60.

837   **Wm. J. Smith**, pauper epileptic from Laurens County, age about 25 years, duration of epilepsy about 9 years, his mind has been impaired for most of the time, convulsions occur quite frequently, sometimes two or three a day, is at times very violent, received July 26 1860, address Jno. T. Duncan, Clerk of the Court of Laurens Co., Ga.

838   **Many Qnarles**, pauper patient from Union County, single, age about 21 years, duration of insanity one year, cause unknown, used occasionally to drink too much, not violent, not suicidal, cleanly, has been confined in jail for a short time, received July 27$^{th}$ 1860, address F. P. King, Blairsville, Union Co., Ga.

839   **Oscar H. Graves**, pauper lunatic from Floyd County, age 25 years, single, native of Georgia, occupation clerk, duration of insanity uncertain, experienced an attack of mental derangement in 1856 in August which continued for some months, when he recovered and was considered well and went in to business for Geo. W. Williams of Charleston, in which business he was engaged, when the present attack occurred, cause unknown, supposed by some to be disappointed affection, by others intemperance, and dissipation generally in a nervous excitable temperament, has been liable to occasional drinking spells for several years, received Aug 16$^{th}$ 1860, discharged Decr. 17$^{th}$ 1860.

840   **Thos. Farnell**, pauper lunatic from Burke County, age 30 years, native of Georgia, duration of insanity four or five years, supposed cause separation from his wife who procured a divorce, frequently stands or sits still for a long time looking intently at some object, imagines he sees things flying in

the air which no one else can see, has a great desire to be roaming about, never satisfied long at any place, he is quiet and orderly, not suicidal, neat and cleanly, not disposed to commit acts of violence, received August 17th 1860, died general debility 27th July 1879, notified.

841 **John J. Burnett**, pauper lunatic from Gilmer County, native of South Carolina, age 32 years, occupation farmer, duration of insanity uncertain, two or three years back became insane from intemperance, was considered as restored and remained well until about the first of this year when from no reason that is understood by his friends, he again became insane and has continue to grow worse, in the paroxysms which occur at uncertain periods, he has attacked different persons and come near killing some of them, acting as he says under the command of God, he is very cleanly in his habits, not destructive nor noisy, it is unsafe to allow him to have anything by which he could inflict injury, has drank none this year, is disposed frequently to abstain from eating under the idea that God has commanded him not to eat, he has heretofore abstained only for two or three days, eating again of his own accord, received august 17th 1860, address James Burnett, Elijay, Gilmer Co., Ga.

842 **Miss E. l. Evans**, pay patient from Florida, age 23 years, single, native of S.C., duration of insanity 2 or 3 years back there were indications of mental disorder, she was then residing in Fayetteville, N.C., the first indication of such state at that time occurred in this way, her mother brother and herself were returning from the Presbyterian Church of which she was a member, when in passing the door of a friend she remarked that she stop and take dinner there, to which no objection being made she went in and immediately after became much excited upon the subject of religion, calling upon everyone around to pray for and with her, remained there during the night and returned home in the morning quite calm, shortly after her return home the minister called in to see the family and upon her coming into the room she exclaimed, let us pray, the parties present though much surprised said nothing, all immediately knelt, and the pastor offered up a prayer as usual, that state was attended with partial paralysis, which has excited occasionally ever since, whenever her health was in anyway disordered or she became at all excited, from that moment there occurred no decided indication of mental disorder until the 15th of this month though she has been at different times since the subject of melancholy and seemed to distrust the feelings of her friends, though those periods were brief and readily dissipated, has had disease of the liver and dyspepsia, her uterine functions are believed to be healthy, on this last occasion occurring on the 15th she is now almost constantly excited, singing and talking loudly (for the bal. of the history in this case see page 220 at foot) [cont. on pg. 220] she has exhibited no suicidal tendency, is disposed to commit acts of violence towards others, is not specially filthy but very careless and indifferent on such subjects, is somewhat destructive, is restive generally and does not sleep, no member of the family ever known to have been insane except an uncle, father's brother, who became insane from pecuniary embarrassments resulting

from speculation in Morus Multicaulus, received August 26[th] 1860, discharged Apl 4[th] 1861.

843    **Miss Catherine Hobbs**, pauper patient from Warren County, native of Georgia, age 40 years, congenital idiot, filthy and noisy, received Augt. 27[th] 1860, died Apl. 20[th] 1861.

844    **Miss Seaby Scroggins**, from Liberty County, Florida, was found wandering about the country, gives no account of herself, was taken up by the county commissioners, received Sept 1[st] 1860, address Joseph Shephard, Bristol, Liberty Co., Fla., died of dropsy July 29[th] 1862.

845    **Mrs. Ann A. Blakey** ,lunatic from Wilkes County, age about 26 years, married, native of that county, had an attack of puerperal insanity in 1852, occurring in a few days after parturition and supervening upon puerperal convulsions, that attack continued for four months when she appeared to have recovered and was believed to be entirely well, has had two children since the first attack, her confinement in both cases was natural and without accident, no hereditary tendency known, no suicidal tendency, is sometimes noisy and quarrelsome, never disposed to commit any serious act of violence, has truck persons about her, is neat and cleanly occasionally destructive, in January last suffered from profuse flooding, she had failed to menstruate for some two or three months previously but was not believed to be pregnant, her health has been generally feeble ever since and her menstruation irregular, both as to time and amount, about six months back positive indications of derangement were observed and speedily became worse, was more deranged at that time than she has been at sometimes since, until about two back, since that time she has been growing gradually worse, does not rest well at night, sleeps very little eats tolerably well, received August 29[th] 1860, address Benjamin C. Blakey, Danburg, Wilkes Co., Ga.

846    **Miss Amelia Ann Hollis**, pauper patient from Putnam County, single, age 30 years, duration about a year, cause menstrual disorder, is a native of Georgia, it is believed that her grandmother was at one time insane, no suicidal tendency, not disposed to commit acts of violence or destructiveness, general health has not been good since 1845 when she had a long and protracted attack of pneumonia, during which arrangements were several times made for her burial, had in 1854 a severe attack of remittent fever, has now had a sort of hacking cough for four months past, received Sept 12[th] 1860, discharged June 22[nd] 1862.

847    **Daniel Curry**, from Quitman County, age 22 years, idiot and epileptic, pauper, about 5 years ago fell into the fire and had his feet much injured, duration of epilepsy since childhood, habits of parents bad, received Sept. 14[th] 1860, address Jefferson Shirley, Georgetown, Ga., died Apl. 30[th] 1861.

848    **Julius C. Pitts**, pauper lunatic from Carroll County, native of Georgia, occupation farmer, age about 21 years, married, has one child, duration of insanity two months, was first observed to read the Bible constantly,

frequently praying when not able to understand what he read, is a member of the Methodist church, was once a Baptist, was excommunicated for playing the fiddle at a dance, has attempted to preach, is at times violent, has frequently threatened suicide, attempted to drown himself in a spring, received Sept. 17[th] 1860, address Mrs. Holland Pitts, Bowden, Ga., discharged Feby 10[th] 1861.

849   **John Tigh**, pauper lunatic from Savannah, native of Ireland, age about 35 years, occupation unknown, probably rail road hand, has only one leg, was admitted to the Savannah Hospital seven months ago laboring under delirium tremens, history totally unknown, being unable to give any account of himself, received Sept. 27[th] 1860.

850   **Miss S. C. Partain**, pauper lunatic from Walker County, age 26 or 27 years, single, member of the Baptist church, duration of insanity nearly two years, is the daughter of a poor man, worked regularly in the field at the time of attack, was attacked suddenly, went to the field apparently in usual health, on returning said she was about to die, went to bed, and has been disposed to lie in bed ever since, a physician was called, she was found to be suffering from suppression, which yielded to treatment, mennorrhagia resulting, she became better, was improving but as soon as she was able to work, her father put in the field, contrary to the direction of the physician, has worked in the field quite constantly since until several months ago when she became uncontrollable, has been disposed to wander and would not submit to control, received Oct 1[st] 1860, address James F. Partain, LaFayette, Walker Co., Ga., died Septr. 6, 1861.

851   **Mrs. Anice J. Harris**, pauper lunatic from Bibb County, married but separated from her husband by divorce, age about 30 years, native of Vermont, is a female physician, a graduate of a medical school in Cincinnati, is believed to have been insane some years ago, on the present occasion she has been insane for six weeks, is considered a very intelligent an well educated woman, writes handsomely in prose and poetry, is believed to have been a lecturer on spiritualism, came to Georgia about 4 or 5 months ago, intending to teach school and practice medicine, is said to have one child about 5 years of age which her husband took on their separation which is supposed, together with ill treatment on the part of her father, to be the cause of her insanity, it is suspected that her mind was affected when she left home, she is the subject of hereditary predisposition, she is usually excited and disposed to be destructive and to commit acts of violence, has threatened suicide, her uncle committed suicide, does not rest well, eats very well, received Sept. 20[th] 1860, address Mr. Jno. C. Curd, Macon, Ga., address her father Mr. Harry Tenny, Northfield, Vt.

852   **Miss Mary J. Daniel**, of Milledgeville, native of Milledgeville, age about 19 years, duration not exceeding three weeks, cause not clearly understood, general health good, usually quiet, but occasionally has paroxysms of moderate excitement, not destructive or filthy, not disposed to suicide, nor to commit acts of violence toward others, slept none

Monday nor Tuesday nights but slept eight hours last night (Wednesday), bowels disposed to constipation, has been under medical treatment since the commencement of her attack, but not bled nor freely purged, received Sept 6th 1860, discharged Feby 6th 1861.

853 **James McGuire**, lunatic from Fulton County, age 47 years, native of Ireland, occupation carpenter, has been in Atlanta about seven months, cause of insanity unknown, has been in the habit of drinking but was not regarded intemperate, has shown no disposition to commit acts of violence, no suicidal tendency known, it is said he had an attack of similar character in Ireland, general health has been usually good, on the present occasion has not been suspected to be insane until about two months ago, has taken work and executed it satisfactorily since, seems disposed to disorder of the bowels, has not slept well for some time, has many strange delusions, received Oct 9th 1860, address Rev. James Hassen, Atlanta, Ga., or Judge Ezzard, died Feby 2nd 1861.

854 **Joseph H. Long**. [no information]

855 **Michael Sullivan**, pauper lunatic from Richmond County, age 38 years, married, has three children, occupation railroad laborer, had a short attack four years ago, got apparently well, was industrious and supported his family, but occasionally has seemed somewhat deranged, but never quit work until about the first of June when he quit work, would not stay at home and treated his family roughly, has eaten very little since then, it is stated that he has eaten nothing for two weeks, has been suffering from disorder of the bowels for four days, probably diarrhea, cause of insanity not known, was probably in ill health, is now very much emaciated, received Oct 10th 1860, address Clerk Inferior Court, Richmond Co., Ga., died Novr 3rd 1860.

856 **John L. Freeman**, pay patient from Alabama, Cherokee County, age 28, married, has five children, native of South Carolina, farmer, duration of insanity about eight or ten weeks, when about twelve years old was thrown from his horse, was insensible for two weeks finally recovered seemed as bright afterwards as other members of the family, received an education, after growing up fell into habits of dissipation, seemed more readily excited by alcohol than persons ordinarily and when under the influence of liquor was turbulent and violent, was struck on the head six or seven years ago with a gum barrel, but was not rendered insensible from it, last spring was struck while lying down with a board three or four feet long and several inches think, the blow was received on the head a little above the temple near the spot which received the blow from the gun barrel, three or four weeks after the last difficulty, was found to be insane, during the intervening time he drank nothing nor was there any manifestation of derangement, has drank nothing of consequences since, has slept but little, has been disposed to eat but little, sometimes has eaten nothing for four or five days, has at this time eaten very little for several days, thinks it wrong to eat, has attempted suicide by hanging, has a brother insane, an inmate of the asylum in Columbia, received Oct 15th

1860, address D. L. Nicholson, Centre, Cherokee Co., Ala., discharged in 1865.

857  **James H. Crutchfield**, from Walker County, pauper, age about 40 years, native of one of the Carolinas, occupation farmer, married, has six children, is a member of the Presbyterian church, third attack, had two uncles insane, had a brother insane, has a sister who has been insane, first attack occurred seven years ago, thought he ought to preach, studied very hard and his derangement seemed to follow his close application to his studies, first attack was manifested by great violence as has been the case with subsequent attacks, duration of the present one recent, but has probably never entirely recovered since the first attack, received Oct 15th 1860, address Mrs. Prior Crutchfield, LaFayette, Walker Co., Ga., discharged Feby 21st 1861.

858  **Mrs. Letitia Grubbs**, pauper lunatic from Fulton County, age 25 years, married, has had five children, youngest now eight months old, native of South Carolina, has had one or two relations insane, one a cousin, has lost four children, last one died over a year ago, duration of insanity supposed by her husband to be seven weeks but thought by some of her neighbors to be somewhat longer, had a severe attack of illness about three months ago, was attended by a Thompsonian doctor, was getting better, able to walk about the house when her husband discovered her to be insane, weaned her child about the time her mind became disordered, has not been violent nor filthy, slept very little for several weeks but now sleeps better, has when excited threatened to destroy herself, received Oct 23rd 1860, address W. W. Grubs, Atlanta, Ga., discharged.

859  **Miss Sarah Phillips**, pauper lunatic from Washington County, second attack and second admission, is more violent than before, is destructive, often excited and noisy, when discharged remained well for about five months, then signs of returning derangement was noticed, she has since then gradually grown worse, received Oct 25th 1860, address B. Glenn, Tenielle, Ga.

860  **Harvey Lanford**, congenital idiot from Gwinnett County, about 13 years of age, received Oct 28th 1860, dead.

861  **Mrs. Adeline E. Bishop**, from Madison County, Florida, age about 30 years, widow, has a child four years old, cause unknown, fourth attack, duration of present attack about four weeks, first attack occurred in the spring of 1850, was insane six or eight months, was taken to Columbia S.C., remained there about six months when she returned home restored, first attack seemed to result from anxiety about her aunt who experienced an attack of paralysis, nursed her, lost sleep, got into a sleepless state which was aggravated by opium, after returning from the asylum was married in Nov 1850, remained well until the birth of her first child when she relapsed and remained insane until Feb 1852, when she seemed entirely well, remained well until Feb 56 when she again became insane, the result of anxiety and distress in the case of her uncle who died, her

child now living was born during this attack, her second child had been born previously without had effect, she remained insane during the last attack, five or six months, began to improve on the birth of her child, remained well until about four weeks ago, her husband was murdered in Dec 1856, which occurrence produced no bad effect on her mind except for a few minutes, she is the subject of hereditary insanity, several relatives of her father's having been insane, but one or two generations back, her own health has been generally good, she has been quiet since leaving home, but before was occasionally excited, violent and noisy, has no suicidal tendency, is not much disposed to commit acts of violence, is sometimes destructive, is noisy at night, does not sleep well, is very thirsty most of the time, has not been treated except to a trivial extent, received Nov 1st 1860, address J. M. Bunting, Madison court House, discharged Mar 15/61.

862   **James R. Thomas**, pauper lunatic from Monroe County, single, age 28, he and his brother William Thomas became insane within four or five weeks of each other, health good, not filthy, but careless, not disposed to commit acts of violence toward themselves or others, always quiet and rest well, received Nov 2nd 1860, address Gwinnett Thomas, Unionville, Monroe Co., Ga.

863   **William Thomas**, brother of James, history same, age 26 years, duration of both cases [blank] years, received Nov 2nd 1860.

864   **Laban Horton**, lunatic from Newton County, native of Georgia, age about 40 years, duration of insanity ten years or more, gradually developed, cause unknown, hereditary predisposition supposed to exist, he was married about fifteen years ago, his wife and himself being on one side of Alcova River and the justice who married them on the other side, the water being too high for him to cross, occupation farmer, exceedingly penurious, has lived very hard and meanly, he has two or three very poor cabins on his place, in one of which he lives in another his family, the only disposition to violence manifested has been toward his wife and children, is not filthy but careless, has many strange delusions, says his wife is a negro &c. &c., is skeptical on the subject of religion, appears to have had lucid intervals, received Nov 8th 1860, address C. A. J. Flemister, Starrsville, Newton Co., Ga., eloped June 19/62.

865   **Abner R. Calloway**, lunatic from Meriwether County, age about 28 years, married, native of Georgia, occupation farmer, is a Baptist clergyman, has not preached for about three years, having about that time exhibited some disorder of mind, commenced to preach when seventeen years of age, cause supposed to be close application to study, sedentary habits, with imprudence in diet, probably suffered from dyspepsia for several years, has been treated for asthma, was quite thin and poor prior to his insanity for several years, has become much more robust and fleshy during the last two years, seems to be now in very good health, insanity was first manifested by unusual news on religious subjects presented in his sermons, has never been violent but is frequently excited, is exceedingly

jealous of his wife, says he has whetted his knife intending to cut his throat, but has made no attempt, is very amorous, received Nov 13th 1860, address Mrs. Abner R. Calloway, Greenville, Ga., or Wm. R. Calloway, Washington, Ga., discharged Apl 2nd 1861.

866 **Walter G. Jordon**, lunatic from Macon County, Ala., age about 28 years, single, lawyer, native of Georgia, duration of insanity about 8 years, graduate of Franklin College, Geo., in 1852, taught school for a time, then commenced the study of law, was admitted to the bar and commenced practice in 1854, has been the subject of involuntary seminal emission, occurring almost constantly, the result of masturbation, has been in that condition since 1852 but says he has not practiced self pollution since 1848, which statement is probably incorrect, has been under the treatment of several different physicians but without any substantial benefit, had a brother who was an inmate of the asylum at Columbia, S.C., no other member of the family known in the past generation, known to have been insane, this gentleman is always quiet and orderly, not filthy but careless, not disposed to change his clothing, no suicidal tendency known nor disposition to commit acts of violence, received Nov 14th 1860, address Ira J. Jordan, Hardaway, Macon Co., Ala., Thos. G. Jordan, Eufaula, Ala., the first his brother the latter his father, discharged 21st Mch 1872.

867 and 868   **Isabella and Harvey S. Mayne**, idiots from Cobb County, the first 15 years, the latter 10 years, natives of Georgia, parents are first cousins, have had four idiot children, hereditary predisposition existing, received Nov 14th 1860, Harvey died July 7 1862 of dysentery.

869 **Mrs. Martha J. Little**, lunatic from Sumter County, age about 32 years, married, has four children, has had six, had premature delivery at six months in January last, duration believed about nine months, about six weeks after her delivery in January had a very profuse mennorrhagia, cause supposed to be uterine disease, no hereditary predisposition known, has for five years past suffered from lewkarrhea [leukorrhea] and prolapsus, her general health usually good, has frequent paroxysms of violent excitement in which she exhibits a tendency to suicide, has attempted to destroy herself in various ways, is not destructive or filthy, generally rests well, is not disposed to eat much, received Nov 16th 1860, address Wm. Little, Americus Ga.

870 **Miss Rebecca Avery**, lunatic from Putnam County, age 36 years, native of Georgia, single, duration of insanity 20 years or more, cause unknown, supposed hereditary, sometimes very noisy and destructive and disposed to commit acts of violence, no suicidal tendency, not filthy but very careless, when a child had an abscess in her ear, received Nov 20 1860, address Samuel Avery, Eatonton, Geo., died June 12th 1861.

871 **Mr. Jno. S. Cook**, lunatic of Newton County, age about 21 years, native of Georgia, occupation farmer, single, duration of insanity believed to be not more than a week or ten days, no hereditary tendency known, has been quite healthy, supposed cause religious and political excitement, has

slept very little for ten days or more, his bowels are disposed to constipation, is constantly excited and disposed to commit acts of violence toward different persons but not disposed to commit suicide, received Nov 26 1860, address Mr. James Cook, Covington, Ga.

872 **Mrs. Matilda F. Mitcham**, lunatic from Sumter County, age about 29 years, married, has four children living, youngest about six weeks, became violently insane a few days after the birth of her last child, in 1853, one week after her marriage she was found to be insane, in a short time she appeared to have recovered but her husband does not think she has been entirely well since, but has not exhibited any decided derangement of mind until a few days after the birth of her last child, she is said to have had an attack of insanity about the age of puberty, after the birth of each child her mind has appeared rather worse than at other times, hereditary predisposition believed to exist, has no suicidal tendency, has not latterly [lately] shown any disposition to commit acts of violence toward any one except her husband, has not been destructive lately but formerly destroyed her clothes and bedding, has been under treatment of Dr. Bailey who bled and purged her freely, certified to pay $6 and her clothing, received Nov 28ᵗʰ 1860, address Wm. L. Mitcham, care of A. J. Williams, Americus, Ga., discharged Feby 2ⁿᵈ 1861.

873 **Susan Davis**, pauper patient from DeKalb County, very little known of her history, has been wandering about the country for several years, staying part of the time at Stone Mountain, has probably never been married, was committed as an idiot but seems to be a lunatic, received Dec. 19ᵗʰ 1860, address Thomas J. Dean, Stone Mountain.

874 **Henry DePeatt**, pauper lunatic from Chatham County, age about 35 years, single, native of Denmark, came from New York to Savannah, went out into the country and undertook ditching on the Ogeechee River, during the past season (summer) contracted fever, had a very serious attack, on coming out of which his mind was found to be disordered, supposed to result from excessive use of quinine, duration about two months during which period he has been confined in Savannah jail, not disposed to commit acts of violence, received December 19ᵗʰ 1860, discharged.

875 **Frederick Greene**, pauper lunatic from Dougherty County, age about 44 years, native of Germany, is a widower, has three children, occupation merchant formerly, for some time past a clerk in a dry goods store, duration of insanity about three months, supposed cause distress and loss of sleep during the last illness of his wife and subsequent intemperance in a constitution hereditarily predisposed, has a sister in the asylum for insane on Blackwell's Island, N.Y., has no suicidal tendency, nor any disposition to commit acts of violence, is usually quiet and orderly, is not filthy in habits, but very careless, received Dec 30ᵗʰ 1860, address L. Barnett, Albany, Ga., discharged & employed.

876   **Wm. A. Choice**, pay patient, brought to the asylum under an order of the legislature.

877   **Wm. M. Pogue**, pauper lunatic from Walker County, married, has four children, occupation farmer, native of Georgia, age 32 years, duration of insanity several weeks, cause probably neuralgia from which he suffered for some months, together with pecuniary difficulty, general habits good, general health tolerably good, is very much excited usually, form of insanity mania, received Jan 25$^{th}$ 1861, discharged March 30$^{th}$ 1861.

878   **James Thompson**, pauper idiot from Fulton County, age about 15 years, idiot and epileptic, is helpless, has been since he was three years of age, had convulsions from the age of a few weeks until three years old, received Jan 30$^{th}$ 1861, address Jno. R. Thompson, Atlanta, Ga.

879   **Mrs. Hannah Fishacher**, pauper lunatic from Muscogee County, native of Germany, age 38 years, married, has three children, youngest eight years old, lost a child six years ago, duration of insanity five or six years, supposed cause lactation and ill treatment from her brother, has usually enjoyed fair health, is generally in some degree excited and often very much so, is usually more quiet when with her children, has a good education (plays chess), has no suicidal tendency, is not violent or destructive, not filthy, received Feb 10$^{th}$ 1861, address Henreich Fishacher, Columbus, Georgia, discharged.

880   **Mrs. Catherine Clark**, pauper lunatic from Chatham County, age about 32 years, has lived in Savannah six years, is a native of Canada, was deserted by her husband in New York, has been living the life of a prostitute ever since she came to Savannah, has been in the city hospital since the 22$^{nd}$ of Oct last, duration of insanity unknown, she had delirium tremens when taken to the hospital, if she was insane previously it is not known, cause of insanity intemperance and dissolute life, is often very quiet and orderly, but more frequently violently excited noisy and destructive, has no suicidal tendency nor any disposition to injure others, she is not filthy but careless, received Feb 15$^{th}$ 1861, address Inferior Court.

881   **Wm. W. Torrence**, pay patient from Russell County, Ala., age about 22 years, single, duration of insanity a year perhaps longer, has become worse recently, his insanity shows itself by singing, talking and excited action, has not attempted any act of violence but once when he knocked his step father down with his fist, has been a member of the Methodist church for a long time, was anxious to preach but was opposed in his wish by his mother, which was supposed to have caused his insanity, general health good, his mother was insane for a short time six years ago, received Feb 15$^{th}$ 1861, address D. B. Mitchell, Crawford, Russell Co., Ala.

882   **Miss Frances E. Rawlings**, lunatic from Washington County, age about 40 years, duration of insanity eight or ten years, supposed cause ill health,

has been in feeble health since she has been insane, received Feb 19 1861, address Mrs. C. D. Rawlings, Sandersville, Ga.

883   **Andrew J. Killion**, pauper lunatic from Gilmer County, native of N. Carolina, occupation tailor, married, has six children, age about 40 years, duration of insanity, he continued to work and supported his family until two months ago, his mind has probably been unsound for a long time, suicidal tendency has been closely watched to prevent his hanging himself, is not violent, thinks he has been poisoned, sleeps badly, generally quiet, habits not particularly bad, received Feb 20th 1861, address Dr. Robt. R. Hunt, Elijay, Gilmer Co., Ga.

884   **John Benson**, pauper idiot from Lincoln County, age 35 years, received Feb 26 1861, died Oct 12th 1861.

885   **Mrs. Elizabeth McGuire**, lunatic from Chattooga County, age about 65 years, widow, duration of insanity many years, cause unknown, is not noisy or violent, is cleanly and quiet, received Dec 2nd 1860, address Zachariah McGuire, Dirt Town, Chattooga Co., Ga.

886   **Martha A. Childers**, from Dawson County, pauper, married, has six children, youngest one year old, is a native of Georgia, age about 35 years, duration of insanity about six months, cause unknown, very little known of her by the man who brought her to the asylum, was brought here claimed to prevent her escaping from the wagon, caused the death of one of her children by pouring hot coffee into its mouth, received March 5th 1861, address John Childers or Fas. Watson, Crossville, Dawson Co., Ga.

887   **Wiley Peavy**, pauper idiot from Taliaferro County, age about 35 years, received March 10th 1861, died Augt. 30th 1861.

888   **Ellen Lyons**, pauper patient from Augusta, native of Ireland, has been in America only four months, age about 21 years, single, duration of insanity supposed to be only two months, supposed to result from suppression of menses, sleepless but quiet, careless in her habits, received March 12th 1861, address Theodore Bridges or Timothy Lyons, Augusta, Ga.

# Names

## A

Abrahams
  Jacob L., 12
Adam
  Duval, 97
Adams
  Edward H., 50
  Elizabeth L., 79
  Julia, 50
  Littleton G., 15
  Mary A[?], 47
Addcock
  Hiram, 59
Alexander
  Jno. R., 53
Allen
  A. S., 40, 87
  Jane, 39, 87
  Margarette A., 29
  Mary Ann, 14
  Robert T., 25
Allredd
  Mr., 86
Anderson
  James H., 51
Ansley
  Elizabeth, 101
  Louisa, 2
Armour
  James, 101
  Jane, 101
Armstrong
  A. C., 100
  Ann, 100
  Hugh G., 68
Arnold
  Bartholomew, 28
  James, 28
Arthur
  Elijah C., 28
Ashford
  Daniel, 31
  Dennis, 21
Ashmore
  Daniel, 1

Askew
  Benjamin F., 15
Atcheson
  John, 24
Atkinson
  James D., 18
  James G., 68
  John, 68
Attaway
  Isaiah, 40
  Majr. Isaiah, 14
Avery
  Rebecca, 109
  Samuel, 109

## B

Backley
  Hannah, 7
Bacon
  Edward J., 78
Baily
  Sofronia, 64
Baird
  William, 71
Baker
  Martin, 33
  W. H., 93
Barker
  James D., 93
Barley
  Jenette, 64
Barnes
  Merrit, 82
  Thos., 29
Barnett
  L., 110
  Tilman, 1
Barns
  Mahala, 82
Barnwell
  Edward W., 25
  Sophia, 25
Barton
  Stephen H., 2

Bashler
  Sarah E., 40
Batt. & Clark, 71
Baugh
  Joshua, 4
Beddell
  Wm. Edward, 7
Belcher
  F. M., 30
Bell
  Missouri J. P., 40
  Wm. A., 64
Bender
  Lewis, 97
Benson
  John, 112
Bently
  Elizabeth, 71
Bernadotle
  Jules, 97
Betts
  Robt, 46
Bigham
  Eliza A., 98
  William, 99
Bird
  George G., 23
  J. W., 23
  John, 18
  John W., 23
Bishop
  Adeline E., 107
  Anderson R., 94
  Reuben, 94
  Robert K., 29
  Sarah, 75
Bivel
  George B., 49
Black
  Ivin U., 94
  Margaret, 18
  Nancy J., 39
  Peterson, 19
Blackburn
  Thomas, 85

Evans, cont.
  Jerusha, 25
  John, 63
Ezzard
  Judge, 106

## F

Falkner
  Henry, 67
Fambrough
  S. M., 53
Farell
  Charles, 15
Farmer
  George W., 25
Farnell
  Thos., 102
Farter
  Bethina, 50
Farwood
  R., 48
Faulkner
  Benj., 93
Faver
  Mary E., 66
Favor
  Jasper, 10
Featherstone
  Elizabeth, 10
Felton
  Richard, 36
Fergurson
  Wm., 24
Fields
  Patsey, 93
Filigim
  Nancy A., 93
Filligim
  J. W., 93
Finelle
  Peter, 80
Fishacher
  Hannah, 111
  Henreich, 111
Fitzpatrick
  Thornton, 7

Flanders
  Madison, 75
Flannigan
  Maria, 44
Flemister
  C. A. J., 108
Fletcher
  William, 11
Florence
  Virginia, 32
Floyd
  Polly A., 36
Fo[?]
  David T., 61
Ford
  Nancy, 77
Forster
  R. S., 62
  Wm. M., 62
Fort
  C. M., 36
  Dr., 3
Foster
  Edward, 40, 87
Fox
  David, 21
Freeman
  John L., 106
Frost
  Malachi J., 33

## G

Gadis
  Harriet, 13
  William, 13
Gailey
  Feinister, 24
Garigan
  James Jr., 22
Garman
  M. H., 95
  Sarah, 94
Garrison
  John B., 70
Garrow
  Wm. M., 24

Gassoway
  Jane, 30
Gavan
  Eugene, 38
  Eugene M., 66
Gibson
  James S., 60
Gilbert
  Spencer, 8
Gillis
  Daniel, 84
  Merdock, 84
Gilmore
  Wm. D., 61
Girtman
  Sarah C., 61
Glassgoe
  Catherine, 69
Glenn
  B., 107
Goode
  Wm. J., 47
Goodson
  John, 27
  Rebecca, 18
Goodwin
  Jane, 73
Googe
  Joseph, 54
Goulding
  Susan, 53
Grant
  Louisa, 77
Graves
  Oscar H., 102
Gray
  Benj. P., 29
  Robert C., 78
Green
  Alexander, 101
  Dr., 61
  Jesse, 101
  Lavina, 21
  Mrs., 71
Greene
  Frederick, 110
  Kenneth C., 80

McBee
  Thos., 18
McCa??
  Hugh, 91
McCall
  Mrs., 73
McClesky, 56
McCollum
  Daniel H., 82
McCook
  Daniel, 33
McCormick
  Frances, 51
McCrary
  Alpheus, 52
  Green B., 91
McCraskey
  Samuel, 8
McDaniel
  Jno., 88
  John W., 88
McDonald
  Alexr., 33
  Eliza, 53
  John S., 93
  Wm. Sheppard, 43
McElhannon
  Frances, 15
McGrath
  Arthur, 88
McGraw
  Arthur, 88
McGuire
  Elizabeth, 112
  James, 106
  Zachariah, 112
McGurl
  Thomas, 26
McHugh
  Sarah Ann, 26
McLanahan
  James, 17
McLendon
  Elizabeth, 10
McLeod
  Christian, 60
  Sarah, 56

McMahen
  Mary C., 81
McMickin
  Andrew, 75
McMillan
  Caroline M., 11
McMillin, 98
  Elizabeth J., 98
McPherson
  Lucinda, 36
McRae
  Martha, 33
  Mary, 8
McRanie
  Alexander, 17
MCrary
  Wm. J., 92
McVinney
  Wm., 9
McWhorter
  James, 16
Melton
  Jonathan, 58
  Sarah, 58
Micklejohn
  T. J., 32
Midlam
  F., 96
Miles
  Elizabeth, 41
Miller
  Henry J., 58
  Jessee, 17
  Wm., 22
Milner
  Jackson, 22
  John B., 19
  Richard J., 17
  Samuel J., 50
Minchew
  Benj., 84
Mines
  Parthenia E., 25
Minte, 14
Mitcham
  Matilda F., 110
  Wm. L., 110

Mitchel
  George W., 52
Mitchell
  [no name], 88
  D. B., 111
  Julia A., 46
  Martha E., 45
  Nathaniel, 3
Moline
  Patrick, 74
Moody
  Catherine, 53
  Margaret, 26
  Sarah, 50
Mooney
  Lucy, 49
Moore
  Catherine S., 85
  Eliza Ann, 60
  F. Carter, 77
  John H., 58
  Sandford W., 60
Morgan
  DeWit C., 44
  Mastin, 6
  Mercy, 75
Morrim, 99
Morrison
  Elizabeth P., 12
Moss
  Almida, 95
  Betsy Ann, 95
  Josiah, 95
  Martha, 95
  Melissa, 36
  Robert, 12
  William, 36, 95
  Wm., 21
Mound
  Martha, 19
Mullen
  J. T., 93
Mullens
  King H., 36
Munnerly
  J. K., 61
Murphey
  Enoch, 75

# Causes of Commitment

## A

abuse
  from husband, 2,
    13, 25, 26
  of her uncle, 101
affection
  disappointed, 2, 5,
    8, 11, 14, 17, 18,
    20, 24, 26, 29, 31,
    47, 88
  disappointed and
    misplaced, 42
anxiety
  attending upon a
    sick aunt, 90
apoplexy, 20, 71
application
  intense, 25
attack
  paralytic, 72

## B

birth of her last
  child, 73
blind, 10, 89
blow on the head, 6,
  34, 35, 36, 37
brain
  inflammation of,
    43, 99
business
  close application
    to, 96
  extraordinary, 52
  failure in, 18

## C

catamenia, 42
  cessation of, 5, 7,
    11
child bearing, 38
concussion, 26

conduct
  bad, of her
    husband, 89
confinement
  penitentiary, 1
  solitary, 11
congenital, 16, 17, 20,
  26, 27, 28, 32, 39,
  41, 42, 51, 52, 53,
  85, 104, 107
congestion of brain,
  21
cutaneous eruption,
  11

## D

death
  of a young female,
    50
  of child, 67
  of friends, 85
  of his father, 44
death of husband, 31
deformed, 10, 31, 54
delirium tremens,
  105
delusions, 41, 54
derangement
  menstrual, 60
  uterine, 57
derangement of
  mind, 68
desire to return to
  Germany, 72
difficulties
  domestic, 29
difficulty
  domestic, 82
disease
  uterine, 34, 56, 109
disposition
  ungovernable, 21
distress, 110
disturbance
  domestic, 101

divorce, 102
dropsy, 43, 46
dropsy of brain, 47
dyspepsia, 82

## E

embarrassment
  pecuniary, 51, 68,
    71, 75
employment
  want of, 18
enthusiasm
  religious, 10
epilepsy, 4, 7, 8, 9,
  10, 13, 23, 34, 35,
  44, 46, 48, 52, 58,
  65, 83, 94, 100
epileptic, 13, 15, 17,
  20, 21, 22, 24, 26,
  28, 29, 33, 36, 39,
  40, 42, 47, 49, 50,
  51, 53, 56, 58, 61,
  62, 65, 67, 68, 69,
  70, 71, 72, 75, 76,
  77, 78, 79, 80, 88,
  90, 92, 93, 94, 96,
  97, 98, 102, 104,
  111
epileptic
  convulsions, 33,
    36, 37, 38
excitement
  political, 109
  religious, 1, 4, 19,
    22, 24, 25, 30, 35,
    42, 45, 47, 49, 50,
    77, 84, 85, 86,
    100, 109
expectations
  disappointed, 74
exposure to the sun,
  100